Lecture Notes on

Medical Microbiology

Lecture Notes on
MEDICAL MICROBIOLOGY

R. R. GILLIES
M.D. F.R.C.P.E. D.P.H. M.R.C. PATH.
Professor of Clinical Bacteriology
The Queen's University of Belfast

SECOND EDITION

BLACKWELL SCIENTIFIC PUBLICATIONS

OXFORD   LONDON   EDINBURGH   MELBOURNE

Osney Mead, Oxford, OX2 0EL
8 John Street, London, WC1N 2ES
9 Forrest Road, Edinburgh, EH1 2QH
P.O. Box 9, North Balwyn, Victoria, Australia

First published (as *Lecture Notes on Bacteriology*) 1967
First Edition 1975
Second Edition 1978
Reprinted 1979

Gillies, Robert Reid
Lecture notes on medical microbiology. – 2nd ed.
1. Medical microbiology
I. Title
616.01   QR46

ISBN 0–632–00062–7

Distributed in U.S.A. by Blackwell Mosby Book Distributors
11830 Westline Industrial Drive St Louis, Missouri 63141,
in Canada by Blackwell Mosby Book Distributors
86 Northline Road, Toronto Ontario, M4B 3E5,
and in Australia by Blackwell Scientific Book Distributors
214 Berkeley Street, Carlton Victoria 3053

*Printed in Great Britain by offset lithography by
Billing & Sons Ltd, Guildford, London and Worcester*

Contents

Preface

This small volume has been prepared in the hope that, in at least some of his lectures in bacteriology, the student will be saved the task of scribbling notes; the text is not meant to be exhaustive as will be obvious from the size of the volume in comparison with that of many other textbooks on the subject. An attempt has been made to highlight those features of bacterial species which are important in their identification and in the laboratory diagnosis of infection. Additionally, brief notes have been included on the epidemiology and prevention of certain infections.

Preface To Second Edition

The introduction in the last edition of small sections on Viruses, Protozoa and Fungi has been acceptable to my students and several reviewers. In this edition my colleague Dr T. A. McNeill, Reader in the Department, has generously contributed three chapters on Immunology which should fulfil further the undergraduates' desire to listen to lectures rather than scribble, perhaps inaccurately, the information which we try to give them.

Similarly the text has been updated in an endeavour to make the Notes more complete.

I thank my wife for typing the script and for invaluable help in proofreading and preparing the index. My publishers, in the person of Nigel Palmer, have been tolerant and helpful in the preparation of this edition.

BACTERIOLOGY

CHAPTER 1
Introduction

The history of any science usually attracts interest from the older practitioners of that science and from professional historians; nevertheless in the history of microbiology there is much to stimulate all microbiologists, including young students of the subject.

It is, for example, fascinating to realize that centuries before bacteria had been discovered, several authorities had postulated their existence and written detailed accounts of how they spread within communities and in some instances had advocated measures to prevent the spread of diseases which we now know to have an infective origin.

There has been much specialization within the science of microbiology in the last few decades; the *fundamental microbiologist*, who is more often a science graduate than a medical graduate, studies bacteria and other microorganisms for their own sake; and researches on, for example, bacterial morphology, biochemistry or genetics are not primarily undertaken with any medical application in view. Antonie van Leeuwenhoek (1632–1723) may be regarded as the father of fundamental microbiology since, although Kircher (1602–80) may have been the first to see bacteria, van Leeuwenhoek carried out the earliest recorded investigation of bacteria in several environments, but his interests in his 'little animals' were restricted mainly to their natural inanimate habitats.

Other microbiologists specialize in the study of the interaction of microorganisms and their human and animal hosts and are termed *epidemiologists*. Epidemiology as a science now encompasses many fields in addition to the study of the sources and methods of spread of communicable diseases, but the basic practice is identical whether one is studying communicable diseases, non-communicable diseases (such as peptic ulcer, diabetes or lung cancer), or even studying the

1

epidemiology of traffic accidents. In each instance the epidemiologist
attempts to relate environmental causes to the ultimate effect with the
aim of preventing the disease by interrupting the chain of events.
Fracastorius (*c.* 1478–1553) may be regarded as the earliest epidemiologist and indeed we still use certain of his words and phrases in
present-day epidemiological thinking and writing; for example, he
described clearly the part played by fomites—inanimate objects—in
allowing the transfer of contagion from one person to another.

Bacteriology made its debut as a result of the intensive investigations carried out by Koch (1843–1910) and Pasteur (1822–95) and the
clinical bacteriologist then came into being; unlike *fundamental* bacteriology, which is involved solely with the bacterial cell, or *epidemiology*,
which concentrates on community phenomena associated with microorganisms, clinical microbiology focuses the attention at the personal
level of the individual patient who is infected and the clinical microbiologist is intimately involved—or should be—in determining the most
suitable antimicrobial agent to treat the sick person. Paul Ehrlich's
dream of the magic bullet, i.e. the use of a single agent which could be
used to treat all bacterial infections, has almost been realized since
the introduction of sulphonamides in 1935 and penicillin (1942), the
forerunner of the many antibiotics now available. It is important to
realize that the blind use of such powerful antimicrobial agents carries
many hazards, not only for the patient but also for the community. A
patient not suffering from bacterial infection may be 'treated' with such
a drug without benefit; another patient may be suffering from a bacterial
infection and be given an antibiotic to which the infecting organism is
resistant. Even when laboratory identification of the organism has been
made and its *in-vitro* pattern of sensitivity to various agents established,
many antimicrobial drugs carry a risk of side-effects, some of which
may be so severe, that one could not justify their use in some cases. The
risk to the community, even when such agents are used intelligently,
lies mainly in bacteria acquiring resistance to one or more antimicrobial
drugs so that resistant strains may spread and cause disease against
which a diminishing number of antibiotics is available.

The clinical microbiologist has a very important role in the monitoring of special units in the modern hospital; certain patients are at very
great risk if they become infected, e.g. the individual requiring kidney
transplantation is treated with certain agents to depress his immune
response mechanisms to facilitate the acceptance of the grafted kidney
by his tissues. These same agents therefore increase the patient's susceptibility to infection and his environment must be as free from bacteria

as possible; not only does the microbiologist participate in the design of such patient-care areas but he has the responsibility of constantly checking on their safety. He is equally involved in the intensive care areas such as assisted respiration units and neonatal nurseries. On a wider front the microbiologist is involved in reducing the risk of infection from instruments and dressings by checking Central Sterile Supply Departments and Theatre Service Centres. The latter concept aims at supplying operating theatres with instruments and other materials which are *sterile* and provided in a fashion convenient for each surgeon; in addition such centralization removes the physically tiring pre- and postoperative preparation of materials for the theatre nursing staff.

The image of the microbiologist, held by many students and too many practitioners, as an individual who blindly examines and reports on material submitted to him is slowly dying; the clinical microbiologist is fully committed to all aspects of patient care, including *the prevention* of infection.

The existence of infecting agents smaller than bacteria, i.e. viruses, had been suspected before the turn of the century—mainly on the basis of epidemiological observations of disease in animals and plants and from which no bacterial pathogen could be isolated; however, the laboratory study of viruses had to await techniques which would allow growth of these agents which are metabolically inert, and thus can only be harvested when grown in living tissues.

Originally viruses were isolated mainly by inoculation of laboratory animals, e.g. ferrets and monkeys, and although in the case of a few viruses such methods are still essential, a great step forward took place in the early 1930s when it was found that many viruses could be grown in the cells of the chick embryo and fertile hen's eggs are used for this purpose.

Most recently, tissue culture techniques have further improved our ability to isolate the majority of viruses.

Similarly the introduction of the electron microscope some forty or so years ago followed by the technique of metallic shadow casting in 1942 opened up new fields to virologists and other cytologists.

The remarkable advances made in virology since the 1930s is now being mirrored in the chemotherapy of virus infections; although numerous antiviral drugs have been assayed successfully in the laboratory the intimate relationship between an infecting virus and the host cell limits the use of many such drugs because of their toxicity to the host which is dictated by the lack of selectivity. However, methisazone has been used successfully to protect contacts of smallpox cases and idoxuridine in the treatment of keratoconjunctivitis caused by type 1 Herpes simplex virus.

CHAPTER 2
Bacterial anatomy

Studies of the anatomy of the bacterial cell appear in many erudite publications; however, in this chapter we must concentrate on the features which have a practical application in medical bacteriology.

Figure 1 illustrates the essential features of a 'typical' bacterial cell.

Cell wall and cytoplasmic membrane

Almost all bacteria possess a cell wall which is sufficiently strong to give each cell a particular shape and its relationship to the underlying *cytoplasmic membrane* has been likened to that which the outer cover of a pneumatic tyre has to the inner tube. The mechanical strength of the cell wall is evident when, under strictly controlled circumstances, it is removed to release the remainder of the cell—a free protoplast—in an intact state. Regardless of the original shape of the cell, the protoplast is spherical and without the protection of the cell wall is osmotically sensitive, so that if there is variation in the osmotic pressure of the fluid in which the protoplast is maintained it decreases or increases in size. Although protoplasts will continue to function as did the intact cell, they do not subdivide.

The cell wall participates in cell division and in determining the spatial relationship of organisms. In the formation of daughter cells, and soon after the nuclear material has undergone fission, the cell wall grows in at the equator of the parent cell to form a cross-wall, which when completed, splits sooner or later with separation of the daughter cells. In many species, e.g. the anthrax bacillus, the daughter cells remain attached and ultimately long strands of many cells are formed since the cell walls remain in continuity; when incomplete splitting of the cell wall occurs the resulting daughter cells remain attached to each other at one point so that a cuneiform appearance is seen on micro-

4

scopic examination. This is characteristic of diphtheria bacilli.

The cell wall and cytoplasmic membrane play an important part in determining the cell's response to Gram's staining reaction; cells which

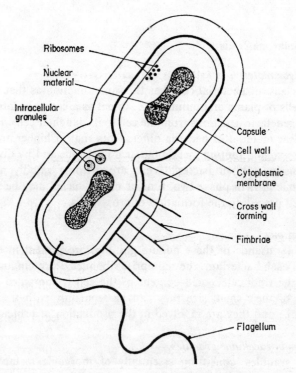

Ribosomes

Nuclear material

Intracellular granules

Capsule

Cell wall

Cytoplasmic membrane

Cross wall forming

Fimbriae

Flagellum

FIG. 1. Diagram of a typical bacterial cell.

are Gram-negative, i.e. those that cannot retain the complex of basic dye and iodine in the face of the decolourizing agent, have cell walls which are more porous than Gram-positive cells which resist decolourization.

Other factors are involved in Gram reactivity and these will be noted later; the cytoplasmic membrane usually adheres closely to the cell wall and plays a vital part in absorption of nutrients into and excretion of waste products out of the cell. Similarly, the cytoplasmic membrane contains many enzymes, some of which are associated with respiration whilst others are involved in the production of cell wall material.

Mesosomes occur commonly in Gram-positive bacteria but are less frequently seen in Gram-negative species; they are convoluted 'warty' structures visible under the electron microscope and are formed by invagination of the cytoplasmic membrane, often at the point where cross-wall formation is taking place. Their function has not been closely defined but they may be analogous to mitochondria of eukaryotic cells.

Intracellular materials

(1) *Nuclear material*
The 'nucleus' of bacterial cells has the same function as that of nuclei in the cells of plants and animals, i.e. to act as a control centre and to pass on genetic instructions from the cell to its daughter cells. However, the nuclear material of bacteria differs from that of higher animals by not possessing a limiting membrane or a nucleolus and by dividing by simple fission. When bacterial cells are dividing rapidly as in the logarithmic growth phase two, four or more 'nuclei' may be seen in a single cell preceding the formation of cross-walls.

(2) *Ribosomes*
Tens of thousands of these minute granules are present in the cytoplasm of each bacterium; they comprise ribonucleo-protein and a large part of the ribonucleic acid content of the cell is contained in them. Because of their small size they can be seen only with the electron microscope and they are involved in the production of proteins.

(3) *Other intracellular granules*
Volutin granules, consisting essentially of inorganic metaphosphate may be present in cells and are large enough to be seen with the compound light microscope; these become larger and more abundant when the cell is in a favourable nutrient environment and conversely diminish in number and size and eventually disappear when the cell is in an antagonistic milieu. They would thus appear to function as reserves of food stuffs; the demonstration of volutin granules helps to differentiate certain members of the genus *Corynebacterium* from each other.

Lipid granules and others composed of sulphur and glycogen may also be demonstrated and their function is probably similar to that of volutin granules; however, they have no significance in identifying species pathogenic to man.

Extracellular structures

(1) *Capsules and loose slime*

Capsules can be formed by certain pathogenic and saprophytic bacteria and are circumscribed gelatinous layers outside the cell wall; in pathogenic capsulate species the capsule is most abundant when the bacteria are growing *in vivo* but the production of capsular material is reduced and ultimately ceases on *in vitro* cultivation. Although capsulation is a feature of saprophytic as well as pathogenic species there is no doubt that in the latter a strain is more virulent when capsulate; this increased virulence is associated with the ability of such strains to avoid or tolerate phagocytosis by body defence cells. Capsular material consists mainly of water with a very low proportion of solids but the latter, usually complex polysaccharides, are highly specific both chemically and serologically, so that type specific antisera can be obtained and used for type differentiation within a species which is otherwise identical. Reactions between capsular antigens and their specific antibodies are thus employed for the identification of strains of pneumococci and members of the genus *Klebsiella* for epidemiological purposes.

Capsules are rarely seen in preparations stained by the ordinary techniques and are most readily demonstrated in films made with India ink when the bacteria appear as faint, grey areas within the clear capsules against which abut the darker ink particles. Loose slime is formed by many capsulate and some non-capsulate species and in the former the slime is often very similar chemically and antigenically to the capsular material; although loose slime is produced when organisms are growing in fluid media it disperses and cannot be seen, but when the same organism is cultivated on a suitable solid medium the secreted slime remains in association with the bacterial cells and the resulting colony acquires a mucoid appearance and consistency.

In wet India ink films made with a suspension of such a mucoid colony the extra cellular slime shows as irregularly shaped aggregates of greyish material varyingly impregnated with ink particles and unlike the capsule, slime lies separate from the bacterial cells.

(2) *Flagella* (Fig. 2)

These are the organs of locomotion in all motile bacteria except spirochaetes; a flagellum is a thin filament twisted spirally and is usually much longer than the cell which possesses it. Flagella are slender, usually 0·02μm in width, so that they cannot be seen under the light microscope unless their width is artificially increased by the deposition

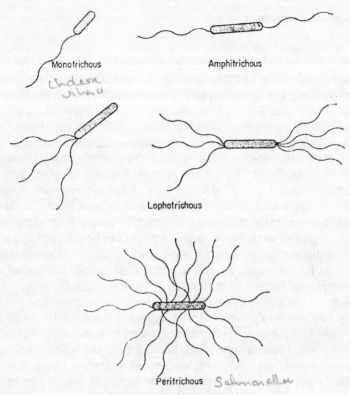

FIG. 2.   Bacterial flagella.

of stain on their surface. In any one species the distribution of flagella is constant. Some motile bacteria are *monotrichous*, i.e. they possess only one flagellum and it is attached at one or other pole, e.g. the cholera vibrio; other bacteria which have a single flagellum at both poles are described as *amphitrichous*. A *lophotrichous* distribution of flagella is one where two or more flagella extrude from one or both poles of the cell and a *peritrichous* flagellar distribution, i.e. one in which numerous flagella are seen originating from the entire surface of the cell, is common in several pathogenic species, e.g. salmonella and proteus species.

Although flagella can be seen with the light microscope in specially stained preparations and also with the electron microscope, their presence is usually inferred *for diagnostic purposes* either by observing motility in a wet preparation viewed by the light microscope or by demonstrating the spreading growth which occurs when the strain is inoculated into semi-solid agar. Flagella consist mainly of flagellin, a protein which is chemically allied to myosin, the contractile protein of muscle in man; as with capsules, highly specific antisera can be prepared against flagellar antigens and this can then be used for determining the serological type of flagellum which a particular strain possesses —this is the basis of serotyping of salmonellae. Motility may allow an organism to escape from unfavourable ecological situations and alternatively to gain access to areas which are beneficial for nourishment and respiration.

(3) *Fimbriae*

These filamentous appendages are approximately half the width of flagella but have no association with motility and occur in pathogenic. commensal and saprophytic bacterial species. They can be viewed only by the electron microscope but frequently their presence can be inferred by the direct haemagglutinating activity of species which possess them. We know very little of their function but since they occur in non-pathogenic as well as pathogenic species it seems unlikely that they have any association with disease production; since fimbriate bacilli adhere to organic particles of various kinds as well as to red blood cells they may benefit the bacterial cell by holding it in contact with a rich source of energy material.

Bacterial fimbriae are a source of confusion in diagnostic serological tests. For example, fimbrial antibodies occur in virtually all individuals and serum from a healthy individual may react non-specifically, often to high titre, with stock diagnostic suspensions of salmonellae if these are fimbriate. Similarly, with certain *Shigella flexneri* isolates type identification may be impossible if the isolate is fimbriate and the diagnostic serum contains fimbrial antibodies because all somatic serotypes of *Sh. flexneri*, if fimbriate, possess identical fimbrial antigens.

Sex fimbriae, or pili, are known to participate in conjugation, but whether they act simply as an anchoring mechanism or allow the physical transmission of DNA through their 'core' is not known.

Bacterial endospores

These are usually called spores and are extremely resistant to adverse environmental circumstances which are lethal for the vegetative cells which produce them. The resistance of spores—many will survive boiling in water for several hours—is due to a combination of factors such as the hard spore-case, the low content of free water and extremely low metabolic and enzymic activity.

Since only one spore is formed by a vegetative cell and on germination of the spore only a single vegetative cell emerges, bacterial spores have no reproductive significance.

Spore formation is restricted to three genera, Bacillus, Clostridium and Sporosarcina, and even then is dependent on environmental circumstances; the fact that the size, shape and position of the spore relative to the vegetative cell are constant in any one species allows the bacteriologist to give a fairly accurate but tentative identification of the species (Fig. 3).

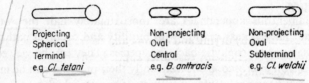

Projecting   Non-projecting   Non-projecting
Spherical   Oval   Oval
Terminal   Central   Subterminal
e.g. *Cl. tetani*   e.g. *B. anthracis*   e.g. *Cl. welchii*

FIG. 3.   Size, shape and position of bacterial spores.

Spores appear as unstained areas in preparations treated by Gram's technique but along with the 'clubs' of *Actinomyces* and members of the genus *Mycobacterium* they share the characteristic of *acid-fastness*, i.e. once they have accepted carbol-fuchsin stain by the Ziehl-Neelsen method they are decolourized only with difficulty, when the preparation is exposed to strong mineral acid; however, spores are the least acid-fast of the structures mentioned since they withstand challenge only by 0·5% H_2SO_4 whereas actinomyces 'clubs' retain carbol-fuchsin when faced with 1% H_2SO_4. Leprosy bacilli are more tenacious and the strength of acid used here is 5% and tubercle bacilli retain the red carbol-fuchsin stain when we attempt decolourization with a 20% solution of sulphuric acid.

Spores, because they can lie dormant for decades, play an important part in the epidemiology of certain human diseases such as anthrax, tetanus and clostridial myonecrosis (gas-gangrene).

STAINING METHODS

Making and fixing a film

Before staining reagents are applied it is essential to spread a film of the specimen on to a glass slide and, after drying, the material must be fixed to the slide. Before spreading the material, e.g. sputum or a suspension of bacterial growth in sterile physiological saline, the bacteriological loop must be sterilized by heating to red-heat in a bunsen flame. The loop is allowed to cool before collecting the specimen with it; the material is then spread on to a 3 in × 1 in glass slide which must be perfectly clean and in particular free from grease otherwise the film will be difficult to spread. It is advisable to keep the film free of the edges of the slide, otherwise the bench and/or the operator's fingers may be contaminated. The inoculating loop is then resterilized and the film allowed to dry in air; it may be held high over the bunsen flame to expedite drying.

The dried material is then fixed on to the slide by passing the latter three times slowly through the bunsen flame. By this procedure not only is the film firmly fixed on to the slide but the bacteria present are killed and preserved. It is wise to remember, however, that the cells have been assaulted by drying and heating and their size is much smaller than in the living state; in any case after application of the usual staining procedures the stained material represents only the protoplast since the cell wall is not stained by the methods normally used.

There are many staining methods available for characterizing certain morphological features of the bacterial cell for diagnostic purposes but only two of these are regularly and frequently in use.

Gram's staining method

Gram (1853–1938) described a technique (1884) which allows a broad classification of bacterial cells into those which react positively, i.e. by retaining the primary dye complex in the face of attempted decolourization, and Gram-negative species from which the primary dye complex is rapidly removed by the decolourizing agent and the cells counter-stained with a tinctorially contrasting dye. There are numerous modifications of Gram's staining technique but basically the method depends on the application of a para-rosaniline dye, such as methyl-violet, to a film, followed by washing off the dye with iodine solution which is then allowed to react and 'fix' the dye-stuff so that it cannot be easily removed when decolourization is attempted with acetone or alcohol. Organisms which resist decolourization are Gram-positive and appear as dark purple bodies when viewed with the light microscope; other species are decolourized and are made visible by employing a contrasting counterstain, e.g. basic fuchsin, and these Gram-negative forms are stained pink.

Reference has already been made to the part played by the cell wall and cytoplasmic membrane in Gram's staining reaction but the mechanism of the reaction is not yet completely understood; it may be that the lower pH of the cytoplasm of Gram-positive cells participates in their tenacity for the primary dye complex but whatever the mechanism is, it depends on the physical integrity of the cell and the presence or absence of magnesium ribonucleate in the cell. Cells which normally react positively with Gram's method will become Gram-negative if their magnesium ribonucleate is removed by treatment with ribonuclease; in any Gram-stained preparation of a pure culture of a Gram-positive species there will always be a varying proportion of cells which are Gram-negative and these are cells which have died before the film was made and have thus lost the power of retaining the primary dye complex. The importance of Gram's staining method will become evident in the chapter dealing with classification of bacteria.

Ziehl-Neelsen's staining method

Reference has already been made to the acid-fast nature of certain bacterial materials and the method used to demonstrate acid-fastness was originally described by Ehrlich (1882). Mycobacteria, actinomyces 'clubs' and bacterial endospores are relatively impermeable to ordinary dye-stuffs but in the Ziehl-Neelsen method, basic fuchsin will penetrate such structures provided that phenol is present and the film is heated; once stained red by this method tubercle bacilli and other acid-fast structures will resist the decolourizing action of strong acids for a time greater than that of other non-acid fast material in the film.

Methylene blue is commonly used to counterstain tissue cells and bacteria which are decolourized by the acid. The differentiation of saprophytic from pathogenic mycobacteria can be made at a microscopic level since pathogenic species are also alcohol-fast and attempted decolourization with 95% ethanol following the application of 20% H_2SO_4 allows such species to retain the red carbol-fuchsin dye, whereas alcohol-decolourization will leach out the carbol-fuchsin from saprophytic species. This has practical importance when specimens of urine are being examined microscopically in cases of suspect renal tuberculosis since commensal acid- (but not alcohol-) fast smegma bacilli may be present; acid-fastness is closely associated with the presence in the intact cell of lipids which, along with fatty acids, abound in acid-fast bacteria since the staining property is lost when the lipids are removed from the cell.

Recently a 'cold' method of performing the Ziehl-Neelsen technique has been introduced since the original method, which employs heat, releases levels of phenol into the air which are much higher than accepted standards.

CHAPTER 3
Bacterial physiology

Whereas the academic study of the life processes of bacteria is now properly the interest of the fundamental bacteriologist, the medical bacteriologist's interests in the physiology of bacteria are very much of an applied nature since he is concerned primarily with producing optimal conditions for the rapid isolation and identification of pathogenic species. Hence in this chapter we shall pay attention mainly to the applied aspects of the subject.

In their life processes bacteria have many points of similarity with higher organisms, including man. They therefore require nourishment and must respire and reproduce. In the same way they respond to environmental factors such as heat, light, sound and other potential hazards.

In the previous chapter we noted the complex biochemical nature of the bacterial cell and when it is remembered that under optimal conditions most bacteria reproduce themselves every 15–30 minutes it is obvious that the cells require almost limitless sources of food materials and energy.

Nutrition
In general terms the chemical composition of all bacteria is very similar, yet there is wide variation in the basic nutrients required by different species; these differences in requirement for cultivation *in vitro* reflect the natural environmental adaptations of the different species and thus their varying abilities to synthesise materials.

Certain non-parasitic bacteria, like plants, are able to rely on CO_2 as a main carbon source for growth and may obtain their energy for synthetic processes from sunlight (the photo-synthetic autotrophs) or by the oxidation of inorganic material (the chemosynthetic autotrophs).

13

However, most bacteria, including all species which are parasitic on man, are unable to utilize such elementary sources of carbon and energy and must be supplied with organic nutrients; such species are called heterotrophs.

There is wide variation in the range of organic compounds which heterotrophic bacteria can use and in general terms it can be stated that the more specific or exacting is a species in its nutritional requirements the more parasitic it has become and the ultimate level of parasitism is of course exhibited by viruses which are entirely dependent on other living cells to provide their food stuffs in prefabricated form.

In addition to carbon, hydrogen, oxygen and nitrogen (which are the main elements necessary for the growth of bacteria) other materials are required in smaller amounts, e.g. sulphur, sodium, iron, etc.; furthermore some essential metabolites are required in almost infinitesimal quantities since they function essentially as catalysts. In many instances these essential metabolites are the same as the vitamins necessary for mammalian nutrition and are frequently referred to as 'bacterial vitamins'.

Respiration

A few bacteria, e.g. the tubercle bacillus, are described as *strict* or *obligate aerobes* since they grow only in the presence of free oxygen or air and alternatively members of certain genera, e.g. those of the genus *Clostridium*, cannot grow if even traces of air or free oxygen are present in their environment and they are spoken of as *strict* or *obligate anaerobes*; the vast majority of bacteria, however, can grow whether or not their atmosphere contains oxygen and are referred to as *facultative anaerobes*. Lastly several organisms are *microaerophilic*, e.g. *Brucella abortus*, and grow best when only a trace of oxygen is present and many such species prefer that the CO_2 concentration of their atmosphere should be increased to 5–10%. All bacteria, of course, require CO_2 for growth but the amount present in the normal atmosphere is usually sufficient.

Recent evidence confirms that the presence of 10% CO_2 along with hydrogen in anaerobic jars (as is easily obtained with the 'Gaspak' system) enhances the isolation of clinically significant anaerobic species.

Temperature

Almost all bacteria which are pathogenic to man have an *optimum temperature* for growth of 37°C and this reflects their adaptation to a particular host. However the range of temperature over which growth occurs varies widely; the temperature range for growth may be from a very low minimum, e.g. 5°C to a high maximum, 43°C as in the case of *Pseudomonas pyocyanea* or over a very restricted range, e.g. 30–39°C as for gonococci. In general, the narrower the temperature range the higher is the degree of parasitism and the more nutritionally exacting is the species.

Bacteria which grow best within a range of 25° and 40°C are termed *mesophilic* and include all of the species parasitic on man and warm-blooded animals as well as many species saprophytic in soil and water. *Psychrophilic* bacteria, i.e. those which grow best at temperatures below 20°C, are non-pathogenic for man but exist in soil and water; certain psychrophilic species can grow even at temperatures below 0°C and therefore have an opportunity to grow on and spoil foodstuffs held in cold storage. *Thermophilic* species can flourish at temperatures of 55–80°C and like psychrophilic bacteria are non-pathogenic to man.

When a bacterium is maintained at a temperature lower than the minimum at which growth occurs it usually survives and indeed almost all species, including those pathogenic to human beings, can survive refrigeration; this extraordinary biological characteristic is invaluable to the bacteriologist since cultures can be lyophilized, i.e. freeze-dried and maintained in this state for very long periods of time without sub-cultivation.

In contrast to their ability to survive exposure to low temperatures, bacteria of any species are killed by exposure to temperatures significantly higher than the maximum at which growth occurs and for each species a thermal death point (TDP) can be determined. The TDP is defined as the lowest temperature above the maximum at which growth occurs at which a species is killed in a given period of time, e.g. 10 minutes. For non-sporing mesophilic species the TDP varies from 50–56°C on exposure to moist heat.

Bacteria which form spores have a TDP of 100–120°C and the most resistant spores are those of *Bacillus stearothermophilus* which must be exposed to 121°C for 12 min before they are destroyed.

Hydrogen ion concentration
The vast majority of parasitic bacteria grow best at a slightly alkaline pH, i.e. 7·2–7·6, although most species are tolerant of a wider range, some bacteria, e.g. Döderlein's bacillus are *acidophilic* and can grow at a pH of 4. Other species, notably cholera vibrios are intolerant of an acid pH and prefer a highly alkaline environment; in the case of *V. cholerae*, media for *in vitro* cultivation have an initial pH of 8·5.

Moisture
There is a wide variation in the ability of bacteria to survive drying; bacterial spores are extremely resistant to desiccation and can survive for many years in a moisture-free environment. Vegetative cells are much less resistant to drying and, for example, gonococci die within an hour or two of leaving their human host even if they are in a favourable pabulum unless the latter has a high moisture content; other non-sporing species can survive for weeks or even months in inanimate surroundings provided they are not subjected to hazards other than drying, e.g. tubercle bacilli can be recovered from floors, bedclothes, etc., for two or three months after they have been expectorated by a tuberculous patient.

Radiations
All pathogenic bacteria are susceptible to the lethal effects of ultra-violet rays whether naturally exposed to direct sunlight or to an artificial source such as a mercury vapour lamp. Of course, the saprophytic photo-synthetic autotrophs require sunlight for their life processes and here again we may note the very wide spectrum of the influence which environmental factors play in the microbial world.

Many other kinds of radiation are lethal to bacteria and gamma-radiation from a Cobalt 60 source is now used to sterilize heat-labile materials, e.g. disposable plastic syringes.

The cultivation of bacteria
In attempting to isolate bacteria from pathological or other material the bacteriologist has to cater for the above physiological requirements in various combinations.

The nutritional requirements are met by providing various culture media; the simplest medium is a *broth*, e.g. nutrient broth, which is a mixture of peptone and meat extract in water. *Peptone* is obtained from the digestion of meat with a proteolytic enzyme, e.g. trypsin and the mixture of polypeptides and amino acids thus released serves as a source of nitrogen, carbon and energy. *Meat extract*, i.e. the water-soluble components of meat, provides various mineral salts and bacterial vitamins.

Since organisms growing in such a broth cannot form colonies, and thus we cannot determine whether the culture is pure or consists of a mixture of organisms, the fluid medium can be solidified by adding a small amount of agar and the resulting medium, i.e. nutrient agar, is usually dispensed in sterile Petri dishes.

Media, whether fluid or solid, can be made more nutritive by adding other materials such as blood or serum which allow the growth of more exacting species. Similarly, by incorporating various chemicals media can be made more selective for a given species, e.g. the addition of potassium tellurite to a blood agar plate prevents the growth of many bacteria whilst allowing diphtheria bacilli to flourish.

In preparing culture media the final pH is adjusted to suit the requirements of the majority of species, i.e. a pH of 7·2, and for particular species, as mentioned above, the hydrogen ion concentration can be altered to assist the growth of organisms which may prefer an environment beyond the normal, near-neutral range.

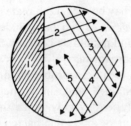 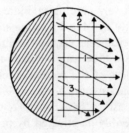

FIG. 4.   Plating out. The standard method of plating out is shown on the left; a reducing inoculum from the well area (1) through the series of strokes (2–5) is obtained by sterilizing the inoculating loop at each stage. On the right is shown the method of inoculating selective media; these media can be more heavily seeded and there is no need to sterilize the inoculating loop between the series of strokes.

When inoculating solid media in Petri dishes it is essential to plate out the material as shown in Fig. 4 so that the resulting colonies will be well separated and if more than one species is isolated then each can be obtained in pure culture for further study.

The inoculated media are then placed in an incubator maintained usually at a temperature of 37°C—the optimal temperature for most bacteria pathogenic to men; incubators are light-proof so that any possible harmful effects of ultraviolet radiation are eliminated. The normal atmosphere in the incubator will suffice for the majority of bacteria but when we are attempting to isolate strictly anaerobic species an oxygen-free environment must be provided; this is obtained by enclosing the inoculated media in an anaerobic jar. After sealing the jar a high vacuum is drawn, e.g. 30 cm of mercury, and hydrogen gas is then introduced and any residual atmospheric oxygen is eliminated either by passing a low voltage electricity supply through a protected electric coil or in more recent types of anaerobic jar the slow union of hydrogen and residual oxygen is effected by a cold catalyst comprising basically palladium chloride.

The introduction of 'Gaspak' for the creation of an anaerobic environment has incidentally enhanced the recovery of strict anaerobes in diagnostic laboratories.

In either instance it is essential to include in each jar an indicator of anaerobiosis; essentially such an indicator comprises methylene blue which can be altered to its colourless state by boiling immediately before it is placed in the anaerobic jar. If on opening the jar after incubation there has been any return of the natural blue colour then anaerobic conditions have not been effected.

Alternatively a biological indicator may be used, i.e. a plate inoculated with strictly aerobic *Pseudomonas pyocyanea* can be included in each jar; if anaerobiosis has been created, and maintained during incubation, then there will be no growth of that organism.

Regardless of the method used to create anaerobic conditions, the basic apparatus must be well maintained and, in particular, cold catalyst must be rejuvenated regularly, e.g. weekly, since the catalyst can be speedily inactivated by products of anaerobic bacterial growth.

CHAPTER 4
Aggressive mechanisms of bacteria

Here we consider bacterial factors which are involved in allowing organisms to attempt to establish themselves in or on host tissues; necessarily these have to be considered separately and in isolation from the host defence mechanisms which are dealt with in the next chapter. However, it is important to remember that the interaction of bacterium and host is complex and, also, that there are still large areas of ignorance not only of the interaction but also of the mechanisms of the two interacting forces.

In contrast with *saprophytic* bacteria which live freely in nature on decaying organic matter, in the soil or in water, *parasitic* bacteria live in or on a living host. Parasitic bacteria may lead a *commensal* existence with their host and occasionally with mutual benefits or a parasite may be *pathogenic*, i.e. produce disease in the host.

Some commensal species can cause disease due often to an alteration in the host's tissues, e.g. *Strept. viridans*, a normal inhabitant of the mouth and throat, is the commonest cause of subacute bacterial endocarditis, but this disease occurs usually only if the host has a predisposing heart lesion and is in a poor state of dental hygiene; similarly pathogenic species may inhabit host tissues without causing any disorder, e.g. coagulase-positive staphylococci are carried in the anterior nares by a significant number of the population, particularly hospital personnel, without any lesions resulting.

It will be obvious, therefore, that the distinction between commensal and pathogenic bacteria (and other microorganisms) is by no means clear cut and that the detection of a bacterial species in host tissues or exudates is not necessarily equated with disease.

In order to rationalize this situation and be able to state, with reasonable assurance, that a particular disease is caused by a given bacterium

19

a series of guide-lines, known as *Koch's Postulates* are often invoked.

These postulates are that before an organism can be accepted as the cause of a disease (1) it should be found in all cases of the disease and its distribution in the host's body should be in accordance with the lesions observed, (2) the organism should be isolated *in vitro* in pure culture, (3) the pure culture should reproduce the disease when introduced to a suitable experimental animal and (4) it should in turn be isolated in pure culture from that animal.

Although there are some infections, e.g. leprosy, in which only the first of these criteria of pathogenicity can be fulfilled, with improving techniques we can usually satisfy the first two postulates; however, since many parasitic bacteria show a high degree of host specificity, e.g. the typhoid bacillus, it is often impossible to reproduce the disease in an experimental animal and hence the last two postulates are frequently not fulfilled. One could, of course, do so even with a microorganism of high host specificity for human beings if man himself came into the category of 'a suitable experimental animal'.

However, there are two pieces of very strong circumstantial evidence which frequently can replace our inability to prove the last two of Koch's postulates; the demonstration of a significant increase in the host's serum antibody level to a particular microorganism is frequently invoked as a fifth postulate and as a corollary a host recently recovered from infection is highly resistant to fresh challenge with the strain causing the infection. The second piece of circumstantial evidence concerns the epidemic spread of a disease when although only the first two postulates may be capable of fulfilment the constant isolation of a given microorganism from each case and the similarity of each host's signs and symptoms leaves little doubt as to the cause-and-effect relationship between microorganism and disease.

FACTORS ASSOCIATED WITH PATHOGENICITY

It must be emphasized immediately that in many instances we still await the discovery or definition of what features of the bacterial cell are associated with pathogenicity.

Surface layers
There are several examples of the important part played by *bacterial capsules* in determining whether or not a particular species is pathogenic; pneumococci freshly isolated from pathological material are

heavily capsulated and therefore relatively resistant to phagocytosis and when injected into a non-immune mouse cause septicaemia and rapid death. If such pneumococci are subcultured in the laboratory non-capsulate mutants can be derived which are avirulent for mice, hence bacterial capsules, by protecting the bacteria from phagocytes, are one of the factors involved in pathogenicity. Similar evidence to that for pneumococci has demonstrated the importance of capsules in determining the pathogenicity of anthrax bacilli, group-A streptococci, Friedländer's bacillus and several other bacteria. No matter how important capsulation may be in determining the pathogenicity of certain species it cannot be *equated* with pathogenicity since some entirely saprophytic bacteria produce capsules.

In the case of typhoid bacilli, pathogenicity is associated with the presence of a non-capsular surface layer of Vi (virulence) antigen and strains which lack this antigen are avirulent; the mechanism involved is not known.

Specialized surface layers, e.g. capsules and microcapsules, can, however, lose their protective ability when the organism in question meets specific antibodies and complement; similarly somatic antigens can have their effect nullified.

Toxins

Many, if not all, bacteria produce substances which cause damage to host tissues; some species, e.g. diphtheria and tetanus bacilli which are only weakly invasive and usually cannot spread beyond the initial locus of infection produce dramatic clinical effects in the host by virtue of the *exotoxins* which they produce; this group of toxins diffuses from living bacteria into the environment and, *in vitro*, can be separated by centrifugation of the fluid medium in which the bacteria have been grown. Exotoxins thus harvested from the supernatant of a broth culture, have so far been shown to be simple proteins, the majority are unstable in that they can be rendered non-toxic, i.e. toxoid preparations can be derived (e.g. by treatment with formalin) which retain antigenicity and are useful as active immunizing agents; the antitoxic antibodies thus produced are usually highly protective to the host. Many exotoxins are extremely potent with a lethal dose for men of 0·0005 mg or less and often have a highly specialized action, e.g. tetanospasmin, the lethal exotoxin produced by the tetanus bacillus, acts on the motor nerve cells. Such exotoxins are produced mainly by Gram-positive bacteria.

By contrast *endotoxins* are released from bacteria only when the cells

die and are not found in significant amounts in bacteria-free super-
natants unless the organisms have disintegrated either naturally or
under some artificial influence. Structurally endotoxins are complex
and their toxic action is similar regardless of the species which produce
them, they are more stable than exotoxins and immunization with
endotoxins produces *antibacterial* antibodies which unlike antitoxic
antibodies cannot nullify or protect against the toxic effects of endotoxins. Both Gram-positive and Gram-negative species produce endotoxins but those of Gram-negative species are most potent.

Toxins are often named according to the effects they produce, e.g.
haemolysin (lysis of red blood cells), necrotoxin (tissue necrosis) etc.

The important role of exotoxin in producing disease has already
been mentioned in the case of diphtheria bacilli; even more significant
is the fact that certain syndromes, e.g. botulism, can occur without the
causal organism itself being present in the host's tissues; here, botulinus
toxin, affecting the central nervous system, may be present in foodstuffs
ingested after the toxin-producing strain has been destroyed.

Other bacterial products
There are several other bacterial products which, *per se*, are not toxic;
but by acting on host tissues may facilitate the spread of infection,
fibrinolysins are produced by many species, e.g. group-A streptococci
and may allow more speedy invasion of tissues with resulting cellulitis
in comparison with more localized surface infections which usually
result with species which have little or no fibrinolytic activity.

Many bacteria produce diffusion factors which are probably one and
the same namely, hyaluronidase; this enzyme, by hydrolizing the
hyaluronic acid which is an intercellular tissue substance, can promote
the spread of bacteria through tissues. As with most 'pathogenicity
factors' there are several highly invasive bacterial species which do not
produce hyaluronidase, thus there is not a complete correlation between
hyaluronidase production and invasiveness.

CHAPTER 5
Host defence mechanisms

Epidemiological and clinical evidence shows that the *age* of the host influences his susceptibility to infection and ignoring other factors which may precipitate infection such as endocrine disorders, e.g. diabetes mellitus or the therapeutic use of cytotoxic drugs, there is no doubt that infection is more common at the extremes of life. The newborn child whose defence mechanisms are being assaulted for the first time is peculiarly susceptible to infection as are old people.

Similarly the *sex* of the host is a factor in determining whether he or she will suffer infection and contrary to the popular belief that the female is a weaker vessel than the male, women suffer less frequently from almost all infections and again with rare exceptions, infection mortality rates are lower in women than in men.

The *race* of an individual is thought to influence susceptibility to some infections but evidence for such thoughts is rare; it is more probable that environmental factors are at work as in the case of tuberculosis where it has been shown that the incidence in Africans living in Britain becomes identical with that of the British community where they live; one example of true racial immunity is known, i.e. although sheep are highly susceptible to natural or experimental anthrax, Algerian sheep are resistant to infection.

Immunity may be defined as the ability or power of the host to resist infection by bacteria and/or the harmful effects of their toxins. Thus immunity may be natural (innate) or acquired, and may be specific for a given bacterial species or non-specific against a wide range of bacteria and other micro-organisms.

23

NON-SPECIFIC SURFACE MECHANISMS

In the healthy individual pathogenic bacteria can gain access only through the skin or one of several mucous membranes and these are in the front line of the normal non-specific host defence mechanisms.

Skin

Skin offers a physical and chemical barrier to bacteria. The *physical barrier* comprises firstly the dead, outer keratinous layer which offers protection against bacteria to the underlying, living epithelial cells and also the thickness of the skin through which no bacteria can penetrate unaided, with the possible exception of leptospirae and treponemata. This physical barrier has, however, innumerable weak points in the form of hair follicles and gland openings through which many bacterial species may penetrate deeply into the dermis.

The *chemical barrier* consists of long-chain fatty acids which maintain much of our skin surface at a pH of 6 or less and creates an environment inimical to many bacteria but there are gaps in the acid barrier, notably in the axillae and groins and these areas, which also have a dense population of hair follicles, may be more readily colonized than the general skin surface.

Mucous membranes

Because of their finer structure these may be thought to be more liable to attack by bacteria than is the skin but the thickness of mucous membranes is enhanced by the mucus which traps bacteria which are then swept along and excreted from the particular tract.

Mucous membranes also possess additional protective mechanisms and those of the various tracts are considered briefly below.

Respiratory tract

The vast majority of organisms breathed in through the nose do not pass beyond the anterior nares and the few which do so are trapped by the nasal mucosa and wafted towards the pharynx by the action of the ciliated epithelium. Very few bacteria persist in these areas and in addition to mechanical removal it is probable that some antibacterial chemical action is involved.

Bacteria which gain access to the mouth are rapidly swept backwards by suction from the tongue, palate, etc. and join those which escaped the filter of the anterior nares; thus many organisms introduced into the upper respiratory tract will be swallowed and subjected to the defences offered by the stomach.

In health probably less than 5% of bacteria which are inhaled pass beyond the upper respiratory tract and those which pass beyond the larynx are trapped in the mucus and then removed upwards by ciliary action and expectorated; the few which reach the lung alveoli are normally destroyed by phagocytic cells.

Intestinal tract

Human saliva has some antibacterial activity but organisms swallowed in foodstuffs will frequently meet their first challenge in the stomach when they encounter the highly acidic gastric juices which are lethal to the vast majority of bacteria. Obviously, if food is chewed thoroughly instead of being swallowed as a bolus, bacteria in it will be more readily destroyed in the acid environment; lactobacilli are commensal in the intestine and would appear to have a defensive role against infection since if they are eliminated, e.g. by broad-spectrum antibiotics given pre-operatively to 'sterilize' the bowel, the consequences may be serious if they are replaced by staphylococci or yeasts which can, under these circumstances, give rise to severe infection.

Genito-urinary tract

With the exception of a small number of staphylococci and other essentially commensal species which can be found around the external meatus, the urethra is normally sterile and frequent flushing during micturition is probably the most important factor in maintaining sterility; the acid pH (5–6) of urine in healthy individuals is also a protection against bacterial infection.

The vagina, particularly from puberty until the menopause, has a most efficient defence mechanism provided by a commensal bacillus, Döderlein's bacillus, which produces a highly acid vaginal secretion by fermenting the glycogen of the vaginal epithelium.

The conjunctivae

The shuttering action of the eyelids combined with the flushing by tears acts as a very efficient mechanical barrier; in addition tears have a very high lysozyme content.

Bacteria which manage to breach any of the surface defence mechanisms summarized above have to run the gauntlet of other equally formidable barriers if they are to establish themselves in the host tissue.

MECHANISMS WITHIN THE TISSUES

In contrast to the non-specific resistance factors so far discussed, all of which are naturally occurring phenomena, an individual may acquire resistance which is highly specific since it gives protection against one particular bacterial species or exotoxin.

When an individual recovers from a natural infection, antibodies specific for the infecting agent are usually demonstrable and such acquisition of immunity is termed *natural, active* immunity because the host's tissues have actively produced the antibodies. Alternatively, *natural* immunity may be *passively* acquired by the foetus by placental transfer of antibodies from the mother.

Immunity may be acquired *artificially* and again this may be *active* when antigenic material is administered to the individual whose tissues then manufacture the antibody, or it may be *passive*, i.e. when antibodies produced in another host are injected.

Active immunity, whether resulting from infection or from administration of antigenic preparations develops more slowly than *passive* immunity, which is acquired very rapidly. When endowed artificially the speed with which *passive* immunity develops depends primarily on the route of injection of the antiserum, being virtually instantaneous following intravenous administration and requiring only a few hours when administration is intramuscular or subcutaneous. However, active immunity, once established, lasts at least months and often many years, whereas passive immunity is of short duration. When passive immunity is *naturally acquired* by the foetus from its mother, antibodies can still be detected in the baby for some months (4–6) after birth. When, however, passive immunity is *artificially acquired* by injection of antibodies derived from animals or other human beings, the immune state is very brief and rarely lasts more than one month since the antibodies are even more foreign to the recipient than maternal antibodies and are very quickly destroyed by the individual.

The mechanisms of specific immune responses are considered in the next chapter.

CHAPTER 6
Specific immune responses

Some properties of the immune system

The immune system is similar to the nervous system. It recognizes and responds to incoming signals and these responses involve interaction between different cells. Substances which provide the signals for the immune system are called *antigens* and the system responds to these (a) by manufacturing *antibodies*: globulin proteins of different types and subtypes and (*b*) by producing a type of lymphocyte which is responsible for *cell-mediated immunity*.

A fundamental property of these responses is the *specificity* for the antigen which stimulated their production. Antibodies and lymphocytes produced in response to one antigen will not react with those produced in response to another antigen unless the antigens are very similar to each other.

Once the immune system has responded to a suitably intense antigenic stimulus it will subsequently make a more rapid and abundant response to the same antigen. Thus the system can memorize its antigenic encounters and this *immunological memory* may persist for long periods of time.

Another property of the immune system is that it may learn to tolerate antigenic signals without responding to them. This *immune tolerance* is important since by using it the system can develop the ability to discriminate between antigens, responding to some, e.g. those foreign to the body, but not to others, e.g. normal constituents of the body (self antigens).

Any account of how the immune system functions must explain these basic properties: the two types of response, specificity, memory, and tolerance.

27

Origins of the immune system

The evolutionary origins of specific immune responses are obscure. Production of specific antibodies is a feature of vertebrates but cellular recognition mechanisms, which may be quite specific, are thought to exist in all multicellular organisms.

It is possible that the immune system evolved from the mechanisms of intercellular recognition. Control of development and growth of tissues in multicellular organisms depends upon the exchange of many types of signals between cells. Since many of these signals are sensed by receptors on cell membranes it is not inconceivable that continuing evolution allowed the development of receptors for the wide variety of antigenic signals which the cells of the mammalian immune system can recognize. This idea has been strengthened by the finding that some important immunological mechanisms are genetically controlled and that the region of the genome concerned contains information which codes for certain cell membrane molecules and is closely related to other regions which are involved in tissue differentiation.

This immunologically important region of the genome is called the *Major Histocompatibility Complex.* In the human it is present in chromosome 6 and four main loci have been identified called HLA (human lymphocyte antigen): A, B, C and D. In addition to these loci there are others, e.g. the I-region which contains an unknown number of immune response (Ir) and immune-associated (Ia) genes. The complex also contains genes which control production of some components of the complement system.

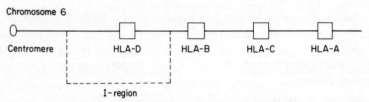

FIG. 5.   Human major histocompatibility complex.

Sensors for antigens

Antigenic signals are picked up by lymphocytes termed *antigen-sensitive cells.* This is achieved by receptors present in the cytoplasmic membrane of these cells. The receptors have a very limited range of antigenic reactivity and to all intents and purposes any given antigen sensitive cell can recognize only one *antigenic determinant.* Antigen molecules are usually complex structures made up of several different antigenic determinants. The receptors of one antigen-sensitive cell may react with one antigenic determinant while other antigen-sensitive cells react with different determinants on the antigen molecule. In order to accommodate the wide variety of antigen reactivity in the immune system as a whole there is a large number of different antigen-sensitive cells.

The reactivity of antigen-sensitive cells for antigen develops without prior exposure to the antigens, i.e. each antigen-sensitive cell is programmed to sense its particular antigenic determinant.

Antigen-sensitive cells are found mainly in secondary lymphoid organs, e.g. spleen and lymph nodes. In these tissues they are in a good situation to encounter antigens since much foreign material entering the tissue or blood is drained into and trapped by the secondary lymphoid organs.

Antigen-sensitive cells develop from precursor cells in the haemo-poietic tissues which are either the same as or closely related to the pluripotent stem cells which give rise to the erythroid, myeloid and platelet lines of differentiation. The precursor cells migrate to primary lymphoid organs where they undergo extensive multiplication and differentiation to assume the morphology of small lymphocytes. In birds there are two primary lymphoid organs: the thymus and the bursa of Fabricius. In mammals there is no distinct entity like the bursa of Fabricius and its lymphopoietic function is thought to be carried out mainly in bone marrow. Antigen-sensitive lymphocytes developing in thymus are called T cells and those developing in the avian bursa or its mammalian equivalent are called B cells.

T and B antigen-sensitive cells have different functions; B cells develop into cells which produce antibodies, and T cells give rise to the lymphocytes of cell-mediated immunity and to lymphocytes which have a regulating function on the immune responses. T and B antigen-sensitive cells have different receptors for antigen. B cell receptors have the same structure as antibody molecules. The nature of T cell receptors is not fully understood but in addition to antigen-specific receptors, T cells also have receptors for some of the cell membrane substances coded by the major histocompatibility complex of genes. This results in T cells having a preoccupation with histocompatibility complex substances; a fact which greatly influences their behaviour.

Cellular responses to recognition of antigen

The responses of the immune system to encounters with antigens usually involve not only B and T antigen-sensitive cells, but also macro-

phages; stimulation and control of responses being governed by inter-
actions between these cell types and their progeny. The complement
system (C) may also be involved in the process.

Stimulation of antibody production involves multiplication and
differentiation from B type antigen sensitive cells. Each antigen-
sensitive cell gives rise to many antibody-producing *plasma cells*. It is
unusual for antigens to trigger this response by a direct reaction with
the receptors on B antigen-sensitive cells. The exact sequence of events
is not fully known but the following outline is in accord with most
experimental work.

Antigens are not completely degraded when phagocytosed by macrophages, and some antigenic material is retained on the macrophage
surface. In this situation it is sensed by T antigen-sensitive cells which
'see' the antigen in association with I-region gene products on the
macrophage membrane. T cells with receptors for the antigen are
stimulated when antigen is presented to them in this way and they
multiply and differentiate into a number of sublines:

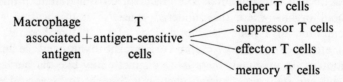

Helper T cells are important in stimulation of antigen-sensitive B cells.
The helper effect is probably achieved by a factor-swapping process;
the complex of antigen and T cell receptor being released from the
helper T cells is picked up by B cells which have receptors for both the
antigen and the T cell factor to which it is attached. Macrophages can
act as intermediaries in this process. The B cell receptor for the T cell
factor is coded for by a gene or genes in the I-region of the major histocompatibility complex. Most antigen molecules are complexes of several
determinants and it is possible therefore for the T cell to react with one
determinant on an antigen molecule and transfer the stimulating factor
to a B cell reactive with a different determinant on the same molecule.
B antigen-sensitive cells stimulated by antigen presented in this way
multiply and differentiate into plasma cells which secrete antibody
molecules with the same specificity as the receptors on the original
antigen-sensitive cells.

Suppressor T cells are important in suppressing the antigen-driven
stimulation in both B and T cell lines. This means that an immune

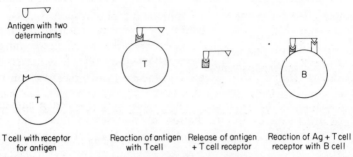

FIG. 6. T cell–B cell co-operation.

response does not get out of control. Usually, the more intense the antigenic stimulus the greater the suppressor T cell activity so that the response achieves a state of balance.

Effector T cells are the subline of T cells which perform the various manifestations of cell-mediated immunity (see later).

Memory cells are produced during the stimulatory response of both T and B cell lineages. These cells are functionally similar to the antigen-sensitive cells from which they were derived and since one antigen-sensitive cell can give rise to many memory cells which often have long life-spans the long-term potential exists for better responses to further encounters with the antigen concerned.

This account of antigen-sensitive cells, their responses and inter-actions allows explanation of some of the basic properties of the immune system outlined at the outset. *Two types of response*, antibody production and cell-mediated immunity, result from having two main cell lineages, the B and T.

Specificity of immune responses is determined by receptors on antigen-sensitive cells. When appropriately stimulated these cells give rise either to antibody-forming cells or effector T cells carrying the same specificity.

Immunological memory is brought about by the production of long-lived cells which in effect expand the number of antigen-sensitive cells available to respond to subsequent stimulation by the same antigen.

The fourth basic property listed was the ability of the system to become tolerant to antigens.

IMMUNE TOLERANCE

Immune tolerance is one type of immunological unresponsiveness.

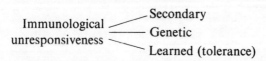

Immunological   ⟍ Secondary
unresponsiveness ————— Genetic
                       ⟋ Learned (tolerance)

Secondary unresponsiveness occurs when the immune system is damaged,
e.g. by cytotoxic drugs, irradiation or disease. In this form poor
responses occur to a wide range of antigens. It is not antigen-specific.

Genetic unresponsiveness has been found in inbred strains of laboratory
animals who are genetically unable to 'see' certain chemically defined
antigens. It is therefore antigen specific; the responses to other antigens
being quite normal. The genes determining this lack of recognition of
some antigens lie within the I-region of the major histocompatibility
complex. It is probable that a similar type of unresponsiveness to some
antigenic determinants exists in some humans but the question is
difficult to analyse in outbred populations using 'ethical' antigens.

Learned unresponsiveness is also antigen-specific but is not inherited;
the unresponsiveness is 'learned' by exposure to the antigens. This is
true immunological tolerance. Exposure to antigen may, in some
circumstances, lead to a specific impairment of the immune system to
recognize or respond to that antigen in a subsequent encounter.

One mechanism by which antigens can tolerize rather than stimulate
is by causing inactivation of antigen-sensitive cells. The complex series
of interactions between B and T antigen-sensitive cells and macrophages
which is necessary for stimulation of the system has already been
described. It seems likely that if antigen makes contact with antigen-
sensitive cells other than through these proper channels then the
antigen-sensitive cells with receptors for that antigen are inhibited
rather than stimulated. Proper introductions are all-important in the
immune system.

If a sufficiently large proportion of antigen-sensitive cells for a given
antigen are inactivated in this way the immune system will be unable
to give a response to the antigen until a new set of antigen-sensitive
cells are made—and this may take some time. Persistence of the
antigen or reintroduction of the antigen in a suitable manner may
cause inhibition of newly emerging antigen-sensitive cells and the

tolerant state can therefore be maintained. Inactivation of antigen-sensitive cells by antigen occurs more readily in the immature immune system of the neonate than it does in the adult. Further, T antigen-sensitive cells are more readily inactivated by antigen than B antigen-sensitive cells. Since stimulation of B cells usually requires the co-operation of helper T cells, inactivation of the T cells means that B cells, although functional, cannot respond to the antigen. This is a rather precarious form of tolerance since it can be circumvented by modifying the structure of the antigen. Thus, if the modified antigen now has determinants for which reactive T cells exist and some unmodified determinants, the T cells can present the unmodified determinants to B cells in a suitable way for their stimulation.

Deletion of specific antigen-sensitive cells from the immune system makes the system unresponsive to that antigen. A similar state, at least in the functional sense of antigen-specific unresponsiveness, can also arise if the normal regulating mechanisms within the immune system which serve to suppress ongoing responses become exaggerated. Strong activity by suppressor T cells can give rise to a state of tolerance, i.e. there is so much suppression that responses cannot be detected.

Complexes of antigen and antibody are also thought to be involved in suppressive effects on the immune system and can therefore contribute to a state of antigen-specific unresponsiveness. An interesting example of this method of control is believed to involve the production of anti-antibodies. Antibodies react with antigens by virtue of complementary molecular shapes. If the molecular shape of an antigen is foreign to the body it follows that the molecular shape of that part of the antibody molecule which reacts with the antigen is also 'foreign' and that it could in turn stimulate antibody production against itself. The molecular shape of the antigen-reactive site on an antibody molecule is termed its *idiotype* and antibodies reacting with these are termed *anti-idiotypes*. Anti-idiotype antibodies have been found in responses to several antigens in experimental animals, but it is not yet known if this is part of the normal response to all antigens and therefore if it could be the basis of a complex network control system of idiotypes, anti-idiotypes—anti-anti-idiotypes, etc.

The importance of the immune tolerance phenomenon is that it provides the means by which the immune system can learn to distinguish normal body components, to which it becomes tolerant, from foreign antigens, to which it remains responsive. This discriminatory ability is less than perfect and a breakdown of the tolerant state can quite frequently occur leading to the formation of *autoimmune* responses. Under some circumstances such autoimmunity can lead to pathological changes, i.e. *to autoimmune diseases.*

The situation previously mentioned where T cells are tolerant and B cells responsive to the determinants on an antigen is relevant to the formation of autoantibodies during the course of some infections. For example, during virus infection of cells virus antigen may combine with normal cellular components. If B cells are present with reactivity for these normal antigens but T cells are tolerant, autoantibodies will not be produced. However, T cells reactive with virus antigens can co-operate with B cells reactive to the virus-associated normal antigens and stimulate the B cells to produce autoantibodies.

IMMUNOGENICITY OF ANTIGENS

From the foregoing description of how the immune system senses and responds to antigenic signals an attempt can be made to understand some of the properties of these signals. The fact that interactions between B and T lymphocytes and macrophages are involved in immune stimulation imposes certain restrictions on the kind of molecules which are capable of stimulating the system. An advertisement by the immune system for the post of antigen might read something like this:

The successful applicant is likely to to be foreign, to have a molecular weight greater than 5000, be of complex structure and preferably protein in nature although carbohydrate or lipid candidates will not be excluded automatically. These qualities will ensure that you have a sufficient number of suitable determinants and are able to maintain good communications between our B and T departments. Preference will be given to applicants who can appear in aggregated form or in association with particulate material since these characteristics are more acceptable to the macrophages in our processing unit. Small molecules (haptens), even though demonstrating highly specific reactivity with a few of our B and T personnel, need not apply.

The immune system is an unequal opportunity employer.

THE EFFERENT RESPONSES

Antibodies

Antibodies are glycoproteins secreted by cells of the B lymphocyte series, in particular by *plasma cells* which are the differentiated end cells of this series. Molecules having antibody activity, i.e. the ability to combine specifically with antigen, are collectively termed *Immuno-globulins* (Ig). Immunoglobulins are composed of two types of poly-peptide chain called H (heavy) and L (light) which are assembled in the manner illustrated in Fig. 7.

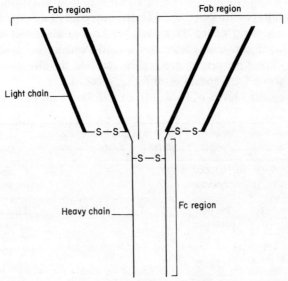

FIG. 7.   IgG antibody molecule.

Both ends of the molecule have functional properties. The end in which both H and L chains are represented (Fab region) provides the combining sites for antigen. The end which is made up of the remainder of the heavy chains (and to which the carbohydrate moiety is attached), the Fc region, is involved in determining transmission of the molecules across the placenta, in attachment of the molecules to cell membranes, in activation of the complement system and in determining the rate at which the molecules are catabolized.

Immunoglobulin molecules bear a variety of 'hallmarks' which are determined by particular amino acids or sequences of amino acids. These hallmarks can allow identification of the species to which the immunoglobulin belongs and the Ig molecules from a given species can be subdivided into classes, subclasses, allotypes and idiotypes. In man there are five distinct classes of Ig known as IgG, IgA, IgM, IgD and IgE, the hallmark for each class being 'stamped' on its heavy

Chapter 6

chain. Some of the classes contain subclasses, e.g. IgG can be sub-divided into IgG1, IgG2, IgG3 and IgG4. Allotypes are minor inherited variations in the structure of heavy (Gm allotypes) and light (InV allotypes) chains. Each individual possesses only a few of the allotypic markers compared with the range available throughout the species. Thus, each individual's particular combination of allotypes is almost unique. Idiotypes are determined by the sequence of amino acids in the antigen-combining site of the molecule whose arrangement determines the particular antigenic determinant with which the molecule can combine. These sequences are highly variable thereby giving a very large number of antibodies of differing specificity.

The five main classes of human Ig have different properties.

Ig class	Serum conc. g/l	Molecular weight	Half-life (days)	Complement fixation	Placental transfer	Other properties
IgG	9–18	160 000 monomer	23	+	+	Cytophilic for macrophages.
IgM	0·7–1·5	950 000 pentamer	5	+	−	First type of Ig to appear in Ab response.
IgA	1·5–3·0	165 000 monomer, dimer and trimer	6	−	−	Major Ig in secretions.
IgD	0·003–0·4	185 000 monomer	3	−	−	Prominent as antigen-receptor on B antigen sensitive cells.
IgE	0·3mg/l	190 000 monomer	2	−	−	Homocytotropic for mast cells and basophils.

Antibody responses

When an antigenic stimulus is given and measurements made of the amount of antibody which appears in the blood, one of two types of response are obtained depending on whether the immune system has been stimulated previously by the same antigen.

In the absence of previous stimulation antibody does not appear in the blood for several days after which the amount present rises slowly to a low level and then begins to fall. This is termed a *primary antibody response*. If the immune system has already been stimulated by the antigen quite a different response occurs. The injection of antigen is followed by a rapid change in antibody levels which usually rise to greater than ten times the amount produced at the height of the primary response. This is termed a *secondary antibody response* and the level of antibody is maintained at a high level, falling only slowly over a period of months. The response can be boosted further by giving more antigen, but eventually a level is reached when increases no longer occur.

The primary antibody response to antigen usually involves production of antibodies in all immunoglobulin classes. The rate of production in each class differs—antibody in IgM form appears before that of the other classes and is usually the first to disappear. In secondary responses most of the greatly increased amount of antibody is of IgG class whereas amounts of IgM are similar to those produced during the primary response. These characteristics of IgM responses provide the basis for a useful type of diagnostic test since presence of specific IgM antibody indicates very recent stimulation of the immune system, e.g. by an infection.

Cell-mediated immunity
Specific cell-mediated immunity is a function of effector T lymphocytes.

T lymphocytes have a preoccupation with major histocompatibility factors on cell membranes in that they can sense foreign antigens much more readily if the antigens are associated with major histocompatibility factors. This applies not only to stimulation of antigen-sensitive T cells by antigen but also to the activities of the effector T cells which are produced in response to this stimulation. Situations in which foreign antigens appear in association with cells are exemplified by (a) infected cells (viruses or persistent intracellular bacteria like mycobacteria or brucellae), (b) tumour cells, (c) grafted cells (where donor and recipient are not identical), or (d) where certain chemicals or drugs combine with cell surfaces. These are the circumstances in which the T cell side of the immune system is most active.

Effector T cells have two principal functions:

(a) killing of antigenically abnormal cells—*direct cytotoxicity*;

(b) regulating effects on other cells—macrophages in particular—by secretion of substances collectively known as *lymphokines*.

Direct cytotoxicity
If effector T cells carrying specific receptors for an antigen come in contact with cells expressing that antigen they will react directly with

the cell and cause its death through membrane damage and subsequent lysis. This cytotoxic attack is, however, restricted to antigen-bearing cells of appropriate histocompatibility type.

Lymphokines
Effector T cells coming in contact with antigen to which they are reactive release lymphokine factors. The biology of these factors is still rather obscure. They do have a number of demonstrable effects, some of which are listed below:

SOME LYMPHOKINE ACTIVITIES

Effects on macrophages
    Chemotaxis
    Activation (increased phagocytosis and bacterial killing)
    Migration inhibition
Cytotoxic effects
Lymphocyte stimulating effects
Interferon activity
Vascular permeability effects

    These activities contribute to inflammatory reactions at tissue sites where effector T cells are involved. They also contribute to the ability of the host to eliminate certain kinds of microorganisms particularly through their enhancement of macrophage function.

Delayed-type hypersensitivity
Whenever a sufficient number of effector T cells are produced in response to an antigenic stimulus, injection of the antigen intradermally results in the appearance of a type of reaction known as *delayed-type hypersensitivity*. This reaction takes some 16–20 hr to appear (hence its name), reaches a maximum size by 48–72 hr after injection and subsequently subsides. The reaction is characterized by a central area of firm swelling (induration) surrounded by a zone of erythema. The induration is caused by deposition of fibrin and by a marked infiltrate of lymphocytes and macophages which are attracted by the interaction between effector T cells and antigen. The classical example of this type of reaction is the Mantoux reaction to intradermal injection of tuberculoprotein in persons sensitized by previous tubercle infection.

CHAPTER 7
Mechanisms of protective immunity

Several mechanisms play a part in the disposal of microorganisms from the tissues. While these mechanisms have to be considered separately for purposes of description, there is much interplay between them, and their relative importance varies considerably with different types of infection.

The main components of the protective mechanisms are:

Phagocytic cells	Granulocytes and macrophages
Accessory factors	The complement system. Interferon
Specific immunity	Specific antibody. Effector T cells

Phagocytic cells
Many types of cell can phagocytose, but two types can be regarded as 'professional' phagocytes: the granulocytes, particularly blood neutrophils, and the macrophages. Granulocytes are produced in enormous numbers (approx. $10^{11}/24$ hr in the adult human) and are attracted from the blood to areas of infection by chemotactic factors. Macrophages, as histiocytes, are found in most tissues and their number can be greatly augmented in an infected area by importation of monocytes from the blood.

During phagocytosis microorganisms are incorporated in cytoplasmic vacuoles and the cells degrade material in these vacuoles by release of digestive enzymes into them. This is achieved by fusion of cytoplasmic lysosomes with phagocytic vacuoles.

The complement system
The complement system is a group of plasma proteins which react in a sequence of enzymic steps. Activation of the sequence can be brought about by two pathways termed the *classical* and *alternate*. The pathways

come together at a point which involves splitting of the third component (C3). The classical pathway is activated by a change in the Fc region of some antibody molecules (IgG and IgM, but not IgA), when they combine with specific antigen. This result in a series of reactions between the first, fourth and second components which results in splitting of C3. The alternate pathway is activated by substances such as bacterial endotoxin and aggregates of IgA with interaction between factors known as A, B, D and properdin. C3 splits into C3a and C3b. C3b remains attached to the original activating complex and initiates a series of reactions involving C5, C6, C7, C8 and C9. During the progress of the reaction sequence a number of 'split products' are released—C3a, C5a and a complex of C5, 6 and 7 which is designated C$\overline{567}$.

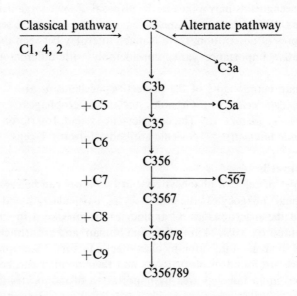

The complement system is relevant to protective immunity in several ways:

(a) Fixation of C4 and C3b to the surface of a microorganism makes it more susceptible to phagocytosis; an effect known as *opsonization*.

(b) Liberation of C3a, C5a and C$\overline{567}$ results in the attraction of phagocytic cells to the area; an effect known as *chemotaxis*.

(c) C3a and C5a have anaphylatoxic effects by causing the liberation of histamine.

(d) Activation of C8 and C9 results in production of enzymes which have *lytic* effects on cell membranes. Bacterial cells exposed to these factors become more susceptible to the action of lysozyme.

Interferon

Interferon is a glycoprotein produced by many cell types in response to a number of stimuli such as viruses and bacterial endotoxin. It is also among the lymphokine factors released from effector T lymphocytes when they react with specific antigen. Exposure of cells to interferon makes them unable to support the multiplication of viruses. This is achieved by blocking the ability of the infected cell to read the message encoded in the viral nucleic acid. Interferon is not virus-specific, i.e. interferon induced by one virus can protect cells exposed to a different virus.

Specific immunity

Antibodies are involved in protective immunity in several ways.

(a) *Neutralization.* Combination of antibody with a bacterial toxin can neutralize its toxicity. Combination of antibody with the surface of a virus particle can neutralize its infectivity.

(b) *Opsonization.* Combination of antibody with the surface of microorganisms makes them more susceptible to phagocytosis. The antigen-antibody reaction may activate complement which then reinforces the opsonizing effect.

(c) *'Arming' of cells.* Some cells possess receptors for the Fc region of certain immunoglobulins. Macrophages can take up antibodies of IgG1 and IgG3 class. Possession of these antibodies gives the macrophage an advantage in trapping antigens with which these cytophilic antibodies react.

Mast cells and basophils have receptors for the Fc region of IgE antibodies. Reaction between antigen and IgE stimulates the cells to release vasoactive substances such as histamine, 5-hydroxytryptamine and smooth muscle kinins. This mechanism is believed to play a role in defence against parasitic infestation. It is also involved in certain forms of allergic reactions.

(d) *Cytotoxic effects.* Antibodies can exert cytotoxic effects in two ways.

(i) by reacting with antigen on the target cell surface they can activate complement which lyses the cell by the action of C8 and C9.

(ii) by forming a link between antigen on the surface of the target cell and a type of lymphocyte (the pedigree of which is still uncertain) known as a K (killer) cell. The K cell causes lysis of the target cell. This phenomenon is often referred to as *antibody-dependent cell-mediated cytotoxicity*.

The immunoglobulin class to which antibody belongs affects its distribution and therefore its ability to take part in these mechanisms. Thus, very little IgM is present outside the blood, most antibody in secretions and therefore in respiratory and gastrointestinal tracts is IgA, and most antibody in tissue fluids is IgG.

Effector T cells are involved in protective immunity:

(a) by causing a direct cytotoxic effect on cells carrying abnormal antigens; important in elimination of virus-infected cells.

(b) by attracting and activating phagocytic cells through the liberation of lymphokine factors; important in controlling the intracellular multiplication of certain types of bacteria such as mycobacteria and brucellae.

It is obvious that protective immunity involves complex interacting effects between phagocytic cells, specific immunity and the complement system. These interrelationships are summarized in Fig. 8.

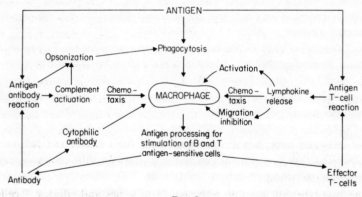

Fɪɢ. 8

This schema emphasizes the central role of phagocytic cells, especially macrophages, not only in the effector mechanisms of protective immunity but also in the role as antigen processors for induction of specific immune responses.

CHAPTER 8
Allergy

Allergy is a state of altered reactivity of the tissues to antigens which depends upon previous stimulation of the immune system by the antigens. It is usually applied to conditions in which the effects of immunological reactions in the tissues make a major contribution to the pathology of that condition.

The mechanisms available for disposal of microorganisms are very effective in many types of infection but their activity may result in a considerable amount of tissue damage. Although the immune system is quite good at learning to distinguish between self-antigens and foreign antigens it is unable to distinguish between antigens which are pathogenic and those which are not. Reactions to harmless antigens may cause as much tissue damage as reactions to antigens which are harmful.

The concept of allergy owes more to the tendency of the medical mind to distinguish between biological events which are desirable and those which are undesirable, usually from the standpoint of individual human beings, than it does to any fundamental distinction between the mechanisms involved.

The two types of immune response—antibodies and effector T cells can be involved in allergic reactions. Antibody-mediated reactions tend to occur rapidly on re-exposure to antigen, whereas those mediated by effector T cells are delayed because of the time required for a cellular 'build-up' at the reaction site.

Three types of antibody-mediated allergy are recognized. These together with the type mediated by effector T cells comprise the four main types of allergy (or hypersensitivity) in the commonly used classification of Coombs and Gell.

Allergic reactions

Type 1	Anaphylactic	}	
Type 2	Cytolytic	}	Antibody-mediated
Type 3	Immune complex	}	
Type 4	Delayed hypersensitivity		T cell mediated

Type 1

Anaphylactic-type reactions depend upon the release of several mediators: histamine, smooth muscle kinins and 5-hydroxytryptamine, whose effects are to alter smooth muscle tone and vascular permeability. Release of these substances is caused by union of antigen with IgE antibody (reaginic antibody) which is fixed by its Fc region to the membranes of mast cells and basophil granulocytes. The antigen-IgE reaction stimulates the cells to degranulate with consequent release of the mediators. Eosinophil granulocytes are also prominent in these reactions. Their precise role is uncertain but it is believed that they serve to clear up the mess brought about by the initial reaction.

Type 1 reactions occur in *systemic* and *local* forms depending on how the antigen gets into the body. The systemic form can follow injection of antigen either as the result of a therapeutic procedure, e.g. injection of penicillin or foreign serum into a sensitive individual, or naturally, by the sting or bite of an insect. The most prominent clinical features of the reaction are dyspnoea, due to bronchospasm and laryngeal oedema, skin rashes, and a fall in blood pressure. These reactions are occasionally fatal.

Local forms of the reaction (atopy) occur in response to antigen coming in contact with mucous membranes. In the respiratory tract the clinical picture of hay fever occurs if antigen is held in the upper respiratory tract whereas asthmatic attacks occur if the lower part of the tract is primarily involved.

While IgE antibody responses are usually part of the normal immune response to antigenic stimulation there is some genetically determined control of the amount which is produced. Some individuals produce greater IgE responses than others and are particularly prone to develop type 1 allergies.

Type 2

Whenever complement-fixing antibody (IgG, IgM) combines with antigen on cell surfaces the activated complement system can cause lysis of the cells. This type of reaction is most commonly associated with lysis of erythrocytes although granulocytes, platelets and other cell types can be damaged in the same way. Antibodies reactive with erythrocytes arise in several ways:

(a) antibody directed against a foreign antigen which is attached to the erythrocyte surface, e.g. microorganisms or their products, drugs.

(b) antibody directed against foreign erythrocytes, e.g. incompatible blood transfusion, rhesus incompatibility.

(c) autoantibody directed against autologous erythrocytes as in autoimmune haemolytic anaemia.

Type 3
Complexes of antigen and antibody which form within the blood or tissues are usually cleared rapidly by phagocytic cells. However, the ratio of antigen to antibody in the complex affects its rate of disposal since soluble complexes formed in antigen excess are much less readily phagocytosed than complexes formed either at equivalence or in conditions of relative antibody excess. Complexes which are cleared slowly will therefore tend to accumulate and they can cause an inflammatory reaction in the tissues where they are present. The inflammatory reaction is caused by activation of the complement system and by platelet aggregation both of which result in liberation of vasoactive amines. Chemotactic factors resulting from complement activation attract polymorphonuclear leucocytes to the area and these cells contribute to the tissue damage by liberation of lysosomal enzymes. Immune complexes may also activate the enzymes of the coagulation sequence with consequent formation of thrombi leading to vascular occlusion and necrosis.

The clinical manifestations of type 3 reactions depend upon where the accumulations of immune complexes are and upon their nature, rate of production and rate of removal. Tissues commonly affected are the vascular system (vasculitis), skin (various rashes), kidneys (glomerulonephritis), joints (arthritis) and lung (alveolitis).

Type 4
Reactions between effector T cells and antigen in the tissues causes liberation of lymphokine factors which attract and activate macrophages and other lymphocytes, and give rise to inflammation. Effector T cells are particularly adept at reacting to antigens which they 'see' on cell surfaces, and they have a direct cytotoxic effect on such cells. It is inevitable therefore that T cell-mediated immune reactions which occur in the tissues result in a certain amount of tissue damage. We are

inclined to accept this if it is seen as a means towards the end of eliminating pathogenic microorganisms, but tend to feel aggrieved whenever the same type of reaction takes place against antigenic material which is relatively harmless in itself.

Reactions of this type sometimes develop in the skin following sensitization by topical application of a wide variety of substances. Such substances, which include some metals, dyestuffs, industrial chemicals and antibiotics are not in themselves antigenic but become so by chemical reaction with tissue cells. The complex of chemical hapten and tissue cell may be strongly immunogenic for T cells and the effector T cells produced in response to this stimulus will react against similarly modified cells. This reaction known as contact hypersensitivity or contact eczema involves redness, swelling, vesiculation and scaling of the skin.

The delayed-type hypersensitivity reaction (Chapter 6) which can be elicited by intradermal injection of antigen into a sensitive individual is another manifestation of this type of allergy.

Allergic reactions, particularly of types 3 and 4, are seen in many infectious diseases and may make an important contribution to the clinical and pathological features of the disease. Thus, the prodromal skin rashes that occur in many virus infections are probably caused by antigen-antibody complexes and the typical skin rashes of measles and smallpox are caused by a type 4 reaction to the presence of virus antigen in the skin.

CHAPTER 9
Prophylactic immunization

In this present chapter we offer a résumé of certain of the practical aspects of prophylactic immunization.

HISTORICAL INTRODUCTION

Perhaps the first recorded attempt to artificially immunize individuals against an infection was that of Francis Home in Edinburgh in 1758; Home attempted to produce a modified form of measles in healthy children by inserting into skin incisions cotton threads which had been soaked in the blood of patients in the florid stage of the natural disease. Forty years later Edward Jenner published his proof of the protective influence of cowpox against an attack of smallpox; the fact that people who had suffered from cowpox rarely, if ever, contracted smallpox had been noted by members of farming communities long before Jenner confirmed the fact by scientific experiment but the excellence of his work rightly allows him to be regarded as the father of modern methods of artificial immunization.

Earlier attempts to protect against smallpox had been practised in many countries and in 1721 Lady Mary Wortley Montagu introduced the practice of variolation from Turkey; variolation, i.e. the introduction into the skin of a healthy person of material taken from the vesicles of a case of smallpox, had certainly been practised in certain parts of Britain long before Lady Montagu popularized its use. Obviously variolation and Home's method of protecting against measles offered no control of the number of virus particles introduced into the healthy person and as the virus particles were fully virulent, modified attacks of these diseases did not always result and severe and even fatal infections were not uncommon in the variolated subject. Home's method of

47

protecting children against measles never attracted attention but variolation was practised until it was made illegal in 1840; by that time it had been accepted that Jennerian vaccination was much more successful than variolation and was very much less dangerous, not only to the individual but also to other people in the community since a variolated person sometimes acted as a source of epidemic smallpox.

With the exception of vaccination against smallpox the agents which we presently use for active immunization against infectious diseases were developed only after the discovery of the causal microorganisms and the invention of methods which allowed the development of safe, killed or attenuated vaccines; similarly the introduction of the hypodermic syringe by Alexander Wood in 1853 preceded the widespread use of vaccines, the majority of which require parenteral administration.

POTENTIAL HAZARDS OF IMMUNIZATION PROCEDURES

As with all discoveries that of the hypodermic syringe has disadvantages; apart from the prospect of injecting material into a blood vessel or causing injury to a nerve whilst administering antigenic substances there is the risk of causing infection unless a *separate, sterile syringe and needle* is used for each person being immunized. Local sepsis at the injection site is probably more common though less serious than the other iatrogenic infection which can occur namely, serum hepatitis; serum hepatitis is transmitted from a carrier or case of that infection by a syringe or needle which is used to inject a healthy person without previously being cleaned and sterilized.

The amount of blood required to transmit serum hepatitis is minute, not more than 0·01 ml, so that transmission can also occur via stilletes used for finger pricking to obtain blood for haematological investigation.

In many circumstances it is more convenient to use sterile, disposable plastic syringes for immunization purposes rather than to rely on a supply of freshly sterilized all-glass syringes; similarly when large numbers of people are to be immunized wider use might be made of needleless, high-pressure jet injectors.

Many calamities have occurred in the past, e.g. because of inadequate control of the production of vaccines whereby live microorganisms have survived in an allegedly killed vaccine; in almost all countries, however, very strict control of the potency and safety of vaccines is now undertaken.

Nevertheless virtually all immunizing agents have potential complications and some of these are noted below; the risk of such complications is statistically small and acceptable when the disease against which protection is sought carries a high case fatality rate and/or is endemic in a community. When such endemic diseases are eliminated from a community (often as a result of active immunization) then the population becomes less willing to run the risk of complications resulting from continued efforts at artificial protection.

Complications of smallpox vaccination

Probably the most common complication in this instance is local sepsis resulting from the implantation of pathogenic bacteria at the time of vaccination or alternatively such bacteria may gain entry after the vaccinial lesion has appeared; the risk of local sepsis from simultaneous implantation of pathogenic bacteria is lessened if the multiple pressure method of vaccination is employed instead of the older scarification technique.

More serious and fatal complications are firstly, generalized vaccinia which occurs most commonly after primary vaccination and particularly if this is delayed until adolescence or adulthood; however generalized vaccinia has its highest fatality in infants under 1 year of age and this is one of the main reasons why, in countries where smallpox is no longer endemic, vaccination against the disease should be delayed until after the first birthday but should be performed before school entry. Also the incidence of generalized vaccinia is lowest in the 1-4 year age group.

A second serious complication of vaccination against smallpox is post-vaccinial encephalitis; it is probable that this complication is not caused directly by the vaccinia virus but is due to another neurotropic virus stimulated into activity by the vaccinial lesion. The incidence and fatality rates of post-vaccinial encephalitis are also minimal in the 1-4 year age group. Such complications are much less commonly encountered following revaccination of the individual regardless of the age of the person; a less important reason for delaying primary smallpox vaccination until the later pre-school years in our society is that the first year of life is increasingly occupied with other immunization procedures.

Provocation poliomyelitis

In 1950 three separate reports drew attention to the fact that a number of patients with paralytic poliomyelitis had received prophylactic inoculations shortly before they developed poliomyelitis and that their paralysis was either restricted to or concentrated in the limb used for inoculation; although this sequence of events might have been coincidental it was soon shown that the paralysis had in fact been provoked by the immunizing injections.

Procedures other than active immunization are also recognized as capable of provoking poliomyelitis, e.g. intramuscular injection of penicillin, although in such instances provocation is usually only noticed when large numbers of people in a community are almost simultaneously injected as in a yaws eradication campaign. Tonsillectomy and dental extraction have also been associated with provocation poliomyelitis and obviously such operative procedures should be restricted during epidemics of poliomyelitis.

The risk of provocation poliomyelitis can be reduced by ensuring that protection with an orally administered attenuated live vaccine is given early in the child's immunization schedule.

Complications of immunization against whooping cough
The incidence of local sepsis following the injection of pertussis vaccine is not known but perhaps the most common complication of vaccination against whooping cough is febrile convulsions with an incidence of 1·2/1000 children immunized with three injections; by contrast febrile convulsions occur in approximately 5% of unimmunized children before their fifth birthday and in association with some infection, frequently of the upper respiratory tract. Thus the risk of febrile convulsions following immunization with pertussis vaccine is much less than such convulsions occurring after naturally acquired infections and fatalities are very rare; nevertheless children with a history of febrile convulsions should normally not be given pertussis vaccine.

A much less common but more serious complication is encephalopathy and although we do not have any accurate measurement of the incidence of post-immunization encephalopathy it must be infinitesimal when one considers the hundreds of millions of doses of pertussis vaccine given in the last thirty or more years; by comparison the recorded and proven cases of associated encephalopathy number only a few hundred. Encephalopathy as a complication of the natural disease has an incidence of at least 0·8% and this risk is very much greater than that following active immunization against whooping cough.

Whilst appreciating the distress associated with post-immunization encephalopathy, this must be balanced against the very real danger of the restoration of whooping cough to its former levels of morbidity and mortality if there is a continuing reluctance to accept active artificial immunization. Such a reversal could easily occur within 3–5 years; this is not to say that an even safer vaccine should not be sought.

SOME EXAMPLES OF THE VALUE OF PROPHYLACTIC IMMUNIZATION

Perhaps the most spectacular example of the influence of active immunization in recent years is that of the dramatic control of diphtheria following mass immunization of the community. Diphtheria was first made notifiable in Scotland in 1889 and during the present century the annual number of cases notified varied from approximately 8000 to more than 11 000; mass immunization commenced in Scotland in 1940 and the annual incidence had dropped to less than 4000 cases by 1946 and to less than 400 three years later. In 1968, six related cases of diphtheria occurred in a burgh in the west of Scotland; two of these patients had not been immunized and died. Their four cousins, who had been immunized, survived; the table exemplifies further the value of immunization against this infection in Scotland.

	Confirmed Cases		Deaths	
Year	Non-immunized	Immunized	Non-immunized	Immunized*
1942	6956	1799	514	3
1946	2122	1024	85	6
1949	272	61	14	–
1959	2	–	1	

* The last death from diphtheria in an immunized person was in 1948 although there were 36 deaths from the disease in non-immunized individuals between 1949 and 1968.

The isolation, in June 1977, of a toxigenic strain of *C. diphtheriae* from a healthy child in the north of Scotland is yet another signal that, at a national level, there is a reduced acceptance of prophylactic immunization and that our guard against apparently defeated infections is falling rapidly.

The evidence of the protective influence of immunization with diphtheria toxoid is overwhelming but in other infections the prophylactic value of active immunization may not be so dramatic and in such instances it is necessary to evaluate the immunizing agent by setting up a controlled trial in a community where the infection is endemic.

In such controlled trials a test group of people to be given a particular prophylactic agent is matched with another group, the control group, which is as biologically equivalent as possible with the test group; both groups should have the same age and sex composition and be drawn from similar social backgrounds. In addition both groups should contain families of similar size and the experience of both groups in regard to past infections should be virtually identical.

Prevention of tuberculosis
Bacille Calmette-Guérin (BCG) vaccine was first advocated as a means of protecting against natural tuberculous infection by Calmette and Guérin in 1906 and the vaccine was used for several decades in many countries although conclusive evidence of its efficacy was not obtained. Controlled trials of BCG vaccine were first undertaken when the Medical Research Council in Britain commenced evaluation of the vaccine in 1949; these trials have shown conclusively that in a country such as Britain with highly developed health services BCG vaccination gives at least a 79% reduction in the incidence of tuberculosis in comparison with an unprotected control population living in similar circumstances.

Another vaccine, the Vole vaccine derived from the murine type of tubercle bacillus, was also incorporated in the trials at a later stage and the Vole vaccinated test population showed an 81% reduction in the incidence of tuberculosis as compared with the control non-immunized group.

Both BCG and Vole vaccines appear to be absolutely protective against the more severe forms of tuberculosis such as miliary infection and tuberculous meningitis.

Without wishing to detract from the value of BCG or Vole vaccination it should be noted that measures other than vaccination have contributed significantly to the reduced incidence of tuberculosis, particularly infection derived from bovine sources, i.e. the creation of cattle herds free from tuberculosis combined with the practice of pasteurizing milk for human consumption.

Immunization against the enteric fevers
Before any evaluation of vaccines is made in the human population they are almost invariably assayed for potency etc. by animal experiment; however, the results of such tests have on occasion been misleading. For example, in the early 1940's an alcohol-killed and -preserved TAB vaccine (alcoholized vaccine) was found to give a much higher degree of protection against challenge with virulent typhoid bacilli in immunized mice than was obtained in an identical mouse population which had been given the usual heat-killed, phenol-preserved TAB vaccine (phenolized vaccine); this enhanced protection of the alcoholized vaccine was associated with the fact that such a method of

preparing the vaccine retained the virulence or Vi antigen and that mice immunized with alcoholized vaccine produced Vi antibodies. Mice receiving the phenolized vaccine did not produce Vi antibodies.

However, when in 1954 field trials of these two types of TAB vaccine were conducted in Yugoslavia it was soon apparent that, regardless of the results of the mouse experiments, the newer alcoholized vaccine had little more protective effect in the human population than had a vaccine prepared from *Shigella flexneri* which was given to the control group in the population.

The group which had received phenolized TAB vaccine had an attack rate from typhoid fever of 6·1/10 000 whereas the attack rates for the groups receiving alcoholized TAB vaccine and the *Sh. flexneri* suspension were 14·1 and 19·2/10 000 respectively. Subsequent controlled field trials with the phenolized vaccine and a more recently developed acetone-killed TAB vaccine in Guyana revealed that the latter gave an even better protection than the phenolized product since the average annual typhoid fever attack rate was only 1/10 000 of the group receiving acetone-treated TAB vaccine.

In these trials of TAB vaccines there was no correlation between the antibody levels which individuals developed as a result of immunization and their protection from typhoid fever; a proportion of people with very low antibody response escaped infection whereas others with high agglutinating antibody levels succumbed to natural infection with *S. typhi*. This latter finding is not altogether surprising since people recovering from the natural infection, and with high antibody levels, occasionally suffer a relapse of the infection in the late clinical stage or in early convalescence.

Such findings underline the need for evaluation of vaccines by controlled field studies in the human population which allow the assessment of attack rates in the protected and non-immunized groups.

IMMUNIZATION SCHEDULES

There are now at least 19 communicable diseases against which a more or less satisfactory degree of protection can be offered by active immunization; fortunately no community requires that the population should be given protection against all of these infections and indeed in some cases only individuals at special risk require to be protected, e.g. those who may be exceptionally exposed because of their occupation. Such 'special risk' diseases against which one can offer active artificial immunity are noted below.

Anthrax   Mumps
Brucellosis   Q-fever
Leptospirosis   Tularaemia

The other infections against which protection may be afforded by active artificial immunization are:

Cholera	Plague	Tuberculosis*
Diphtheria*	Poliomyelitis*	Typhoid fever
Influenza	Rubella*	Typhus fever
Measles*	Smallpox*	Yellow fever
Pertussis*	Tetanus*	

Those infections against which children in Britain still require protection are asterisked but the above list should also remind us that diseases such as cholera, plague and typhus fever rampaged through this country until relatively recently and were driven out by measures such as improved sanitation and safe water supplies; the continuing presence of these same infections in other countries underlines the need for such measures as well as the practice of preventive medicine.

Recommendations regarding which vaccines should be offered to a community and the priority in which vaccines are given can only be made with a knowledge of the morbidity and mortality rates of the several diseases; obviously since whooping cough, although uncommon in the first six months of life, is restricted in its lethality to the first year then pertussis vaccine must be given precedence in Britain. Fortunately this vaccine can be combined with diphtheria toxoid and tetanus toxoid so that the young infant can be simultaneously protected against three diseases.

The following immunization schedule is that suggested for countries such as Britain where the Public Health medical services are well developed.

IMMUNIZATION SCHEDULE

Age	Visit	Vaccine	Time interval
3–12 months	1	Triple* & oral polio	
	2	,, ,, ,, ,,	6 weeks
	3	,, ,, ,, ,,	4–6 months
2–4 years	4	Smallpox & measles†	
5 years	5	Dip./Tet. & oral polio	
9 years	6	Dip./Tet. & smallpox	
15 years	7	BCG	

* Triple vaccine comprises diphtheria, pertussis and tetanus antigens.

† An interval of at least 3 weeks must separate these procedures from each other and from the administration of any other live vaccine.

All girls aged 11–13 years should be offered rubella vaccine whether or not there is a past history of infection.

Following on the programme, mounted by WHO, for the global eradication of smallpox an official decision recommended that primary smallpox vaccination need no longer be undertaken in childhood; there are some who do not agree with this recommendation since *inter alia* the risk of complications following primary vaccination in childhood are very small compared with equivalent risks when primary vaccination is made in adolescence or adulthood. Certainly there are professional groups, e.g. medical and nursing personnel, ambulance men and laboratory workers, who must continue to receive such protection and it would seem a wise policy still to recommend primary vaccination in childhood to avoid unnecessary complications when such vaccination is delayed until adulthood.

Reference has already been made to the need for introducing and continuing other methods of disease prevention such as the provision of safe water supplies and the production of milk free from bovine tubercle bacilli; similarly the education of mothers regarding such matters as the preparation of safe milk feeds for artificially fed infants can do much to protect babies against infantile gastroenteritis which still makes a significant contribution to infant mortality rates in many developing countries.

Whilst such countries are faced with serious problems of health education Britain and other more sophisticated communities are similarly placed in regard to persuading mothers to have their children fully immunized; while it remains impossible to combine all vaccines then a minimum of four visits are required for immunization purposes in the child's pre-school days and such a programme may become impracticable for the mother with a young family and a recent addition thereto.

Another reason for constantly reminding mothers of the need to have their children protected against certain infections is that the very success of active immunization procedures has led to the virtual elimination of some infections, e.g. diphtheria in this country so that the young mother of today is aware of the potentially lethal nature of such diseases only from family folk-lore.

CHAPTER 10
Serology

Serology is the study of the reaction between antigens and antibodies. Wide use is made of these reactions in diagnostic procedures.

(1) *Skin Tests*
There are several tests available where the principle is that a prepared antigen is injected intradermally in safe dosage and if the individual does not possess antibodies specific to the antigen, i.e. he has no specific acquired immunity, a skin response occurs, e.g. erythema with or without local oedema. Individuals who have acquired immunity will not show a response since the antigenic material is neutralized by the specific antibody in their tissues.

(2) *Laboratory tests*
In vitro methods have been devised which allow us to observe the specificity of reaction between antigens and their antibodies. Obviously such tests can be used in two ways, firstly, if we prepare antisera specific for particular bacteria or bacterial components, these prepared or stock antisera can then be used to identify bacteria isolated from pathological material. Alternatively, by maintaining stock strains of fully identified bacteria, we can use these to detect specific antibodies in samples of human serum.

Less commonly, laboratory animals can be used for the *in vivo* demonstration of antigen-antibody reactions, e.g. in determining whether a diphtheria bacillus isolated from an individual is capable of producing exotoxin (see Chapter 16).

IN VITRO REACTIONS

AGGLUTINATION

Agglutination occurs where the test antigen comprises a suspension of intact bacterial cells and these clump together in the presence of specific antibody and the aggregated cells then form a deposit in the test-tube and the supernatant fluid, which was originally turbid, becomes clear.

The phrase 'agglutination test' is almost synonymous with the Widal test employed in detecting antibodies specific for salmonellae because although agglutination techniques are used to detect antibodies specific for bacteria in other genera, the Widal test is far and away the most frequently performed.

Widal test

As with most other *in vitro* serological tests the Widal test is *quantitative*. A series of six tubes is set up so that each contains an identical unit volume of patient's serum but in doubling dilutions from 1 in 15 to 1 in 480 and then to each tube is added a unit volume of stock bacillary suspension so that the final serial dilutions of patient's serum are from 1 in 30 to 1 in 960. A seventh tube containing only a unit volume of stock bacillary suspension and an equal amount of sterile physiological saline is included in the test to ensure that the stock suspension is not auto-agglutinable.

After thorough mixing, the contents of each tube are transferred by individual pipettes to agglutination tubes which are incubated at 37°C for 4 hr; thereafter the antibody titre of the patient's serum is taken as that in the tube containing the highest dilution of serum in which agglutination is noted.

If a formalized bacterial suspension is used in the test then the serum agglutinins which cause agglutination are flagellar antibodies, and similarly an alcoholized suspension detects somatic antibodies. Thus by parallel testing of separate aliquots of the patient's serum with formalized and alcoholized bacillary suspensions one can obtain additional information which aids interpretation of the result.

Interpretation of Widal test

Many individuals possess antibodies to certain salmonellae and yet have never suffered infection by such species; such *normal antibody levels* vary with the country in which the person lives and even vary in diffe.ent parts of one country. In Britain the following titres are accepted as being within normal limits; for *Salmonella typhi* and *Salmonella paratyphi B*, H (flagellar) agglutination = 1 in 30 and O (somatic) agglutination = 1 in 50; for *Salmonella paratyphi A* and *C* both H and O reactions = 1 in 10.

Prior immunization with TAB vaccine can cause confusion in interpretation of results since titres, particularly of H agglutinins, may persist for many months after immunization. In such cases, doubt as to the significance of the result can often be resolved by repeating the test on a second serum sample taken 7–10 days after the first. If the titre of the second specimen is the same as that of the first then it is unlikely that the individual is suffering from active infection. However, even a definite rise in titre does not imply active infection since the rise may be caused by non-specific factors, e.g. a febrile, non-enteric condition, in which case the titre of the serum rapidly reverts to its original level when the non-enteric infection ceases.

Certain non-specific antigens, e.g. fimbrial antigens may be present in the test suspension and react with fimbrial antibodies in the patient's serum, often to very high titre, without significance. Obviously test suspensions must be devoid of such non-specific antigens.

PRECIPITATION

If instead of using intact bacterial cells we employ an extract of the cells as a colloidal solution and, in a tube, layer the antigen over its specific antiserum then precipitation occurs at the interface. The most common use of this method in diagnostic laboratories involves the determination of the group-specificity of β-haemolytic streptococci. After chemical extraction of the group-specific polysaccharide antigen from a culture it is layered into several tubes each containing equal volumes of various group-specific antisera and within a few minutes dense precipitation will occur at the interface of the tube containing the antiserum specific for the particular antigenic extract.

For research purposes gel-diffusion tests may be performed in Petri dishes or other suitable containers. Several variations of the basic technique are available but they all depend on using an agar gel which allows antigen and antibody to diffuse towards one another from wells or holes punched out of the agar and when specific components of each meet in the proper ratio, lines of precipitation appear in the agar. Such a method can be used to detect toxigenicity in diphtheria bacilli and can be used in place of *in-vivo* animal experiments.

BACTERIOLYSIS

When, in the presence of normal serum complement, specific anti-bacterial antibody meets the bacterial cells which stimulated its formation the latter are lysed; this can be demonstrated *in vitro* by noting the elimination of turbidity in a tube test and also *in vivo* (Pfeiffer's reaction). In the latter instance a guinea-pig receives an intraperitoneal injection of cholera vibrios along with anticholera serum previously heated to destroy its natural complement. By withdrawing fluid from the peritoneum at 10 or 15 min intervals one can note the vibrios undergoing lysis and within an hour or two none will be detectable. Here the natural guinea-pig complement has acted in concert with the injected antibody.

Complement is a group of proteins which occur naturally in the serum of individuals whether or not the person is immune to a disease or diseases. It deteriorates rapidly once serum has been withdrawn from the individual and can be speedily inactivated, without altering any antibody content, by heating the serum at 55°C for 30 min.

Bacteriolysis tests, as an indicator of specificity of antigen and antibody, are not used for diagnostic purposes but the analogous lysis of red blood cells (RBC) by specific haemolytic antiserum is made use of as an indicator system in complement-fixation tests; as in bacteriolysis, haemolysis of the target cell cannot be effected by complement alone or by the haemolytic antiserum if its natural complement has been inactivated. Hence, by mixing red cells with *heated* specific haemolytic antiserum one has a sensitized system which will remain unaltered in the absence of complement but which will show lysis of the RBC if complement is added.

COMPLEMENT FIXATION

If to a bacterial antigen one adds *heated* specific antiserum and a measured amount of complement from another source (usually guinea-pig serum) then when the antigen and antibody unite they bind or fix the complement, however the fixation of the complement is not visually detectable. One must then add a volume of sensitized RBC and since the complement is not available to complete the sensitized system there is no lysis of RBC and the complement-fixation test is positive, i.e. the heated serum contained specific antibody for the antigen in the original mixture. Conversely, if the stock antigen had no specific counterpart in the heated serum they would not unite and hence the complement would be free to complete the sensitized RBC system and when the latter is added lysis would occur, i.e. a negative complement-fixation test.

Although complement-fixation tests are widely used in other branches of microbiology, e.g. virology, they are not widely used in diagnostic bacteriology laboratories and indeed, the phrase 'complement-fixation test' is almost synonymous with the Wassermann test used in the sero-diagnosis of syphilis.

The Wassermann test is performed quantitatively, thus one can follow the results of treating the disease since strongly positive re-actions with patient's serum taken before therapy become progressively weaker as infection is eliminated. As with the interpretation of Widal test results various factors other than syphilitic infection may give a positive finding, e.g. in tropical countries the sera of patients suffering from yaws, which is a non-venereal treponemal infection, will react positively as will a proportion of cases of malaria.

In temperate zones false positive Wassermann reactions occur oc-casionally in patients suffering from collagen diseases and from certain infections, particularly of the respiratory tract. However, such reactions are short-lived and negative test results are found shortly after the causal, non-syphilitic condition is cured.

The sera of pregnant women occasionally show false positive Wasser-mann reactions and thus alternative tests are employed to confirm whether or not the individual is suffering from syphilis.

OPSONIZATION

Opsonins occur naturally in normal serum and they can alter the sur-face characteristics of bacteria which are then more susceptible to phagocytosis. Naturally occurring opsonins are thermolabile in contrast to opsonins found in the serum as a result of infection. These thermo-stable immune opsonins also facilitate phagocytosis of the bacterial cells which stimulated their formation.

Tests of opsonocytophagic activity in sera are technically difficult and not statistically reliable so that they are no longer in general use. They were performed by estimating the average number of bacteria ingested by phagocytes in the presence of a patient's serum and com-paring this with the number of the same bacteria phagocytosed in a non-immune control serum.

NEUTRALIZATION TESTS

In cases where a suitable laboratory animal is susceptible to infection with a bacterium or alternatively reacts to a bacterial toxin, then the specific antibacterial antibody or antitoxin should protect the animal. In such tests a pair of animals is used and these should be as identical as possible, e.g. in age, sex, weight etc.; one is 'protected' (the control animal) by administration of antibody before it and its unprotected companion (the test animal) receive identical challenge doses of the antigen.

It may be that both animals show no response when challenged or both suffer ill effects. However, if the test animal shows pathognomonic evidence for the particular challenge material whereas the control animal suffers no effect, then we conclude that the antigen used to challenge the pair is specific for the antibody used to protect the control animal.

Obviously neutralization tests can also be used to detect 'unknown' antibody if one challenges with a known antigen and such tests can be made quantitative by using a series of biologically equivalent animals and, whilst maintaining a constant concentration of either antigen or antibody, one varies the concentration of the other reagent. This latter is the basis of assaying the potency of immunizing agents.

CHAPTER 11
Sources and methods of spread of infection

An understanding of the sources and methods of spread of infection allows intelligent action to be taken, aimed at reducing the risk of infection in a susceptible individual and interrupting epidemic spread in a community.

The sources of infection for man are *other human beings, animals* and, in a few instances, the *soil*; human infections acquired from animal sources are called zoonoses.

Man as a source of infection
Most human infections are acquired from other humans and the source may be a sick person or a carrier. The severity of the infection in the sick individual does not necessarily indicate how dangerous he is to other people; indeed, a patient suffering from a mild infection often continues at work and can therefore disseminate the infecting organism to many more people than if his illness were severe enough to require isolation or bed-rest at home or in hospital.

Carriers may be defined as individuals who are found to be excreting pathogenic microorganisms but are not, at the time, suffering any disease; there are two kinds of carrier, the *convalescent* carrier is one who has recovered from an infection but continues to excrete the causal organism. Convalescent carriers are divided into temporary (transient) carriers and chronic (permanent) carriers depending on the duration of excretion after clinical recovery; the time interval after which a temporary carrier is regarded as becoming a permanent carrier varies with different diseases and the division is entirely arbitrary. In contrast to the convalescent carrier a person may be a *healthy* carrier, i.e. to the best of everyone's knowledge he has never suffered clinical infection caused by the organism he is excreting.

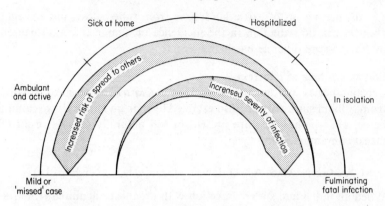

FIG. 9.   Severity of infection in the individual is inversely related to his potential
as a source of infection.

In theory at least, the convalescent carrier should be less likely to
act as a source of infection for other susceptible individuals since he is
a recognized carrier. By contrast, the healthy carrier is not recognized
as a potential source of infection until he has been detected incidentally
during investigation of a particular epidemic or alternatively when a
carrier survey is carried out.

Human carriers are a frequent source of many infections and may
be a greater risk to other men since their carrier state may not have
been recognized. In certain circumstances and contrary to what might
be thought, the chronic carrier is less of a risk as a source of infection
than the temporary carrier, since the species which he is excreting may
lose its pathogenicity over a period of time. For example, group-A
streptococci produce reducing amounts of M antigen as carriage continues, and since this type-specific protein antigen is an important
factor (perhaps the most important) in determining pathogenicity in
such species we can explain why relatively few fresh cases can be traced
to chronic carriers.

Animals as a source of infection
In most zoonoses it is unusual for the infected human being to act as
a source for other men. Both domestic and wild animals act as sources
and in either instance the animal may be sick or may be a carrier.
Obviously there is an occupational risk of acquiring certain zoonoses,
e.g. farmers and veterinary surgeons and abattoir workers have a continuing and closer involvement with many animals than the general
population which may be protected by some legally required process,

e.g. the setting up of cattle herds free from tuberculosis has brought about a drastic reduction in the incidence of human infection caused by bovine-type tubercle bacilli.

Soil as a source of infection
Certain species, particularly of the genus *Clostridium*, can be isolated from soil but since they are also excreted by man and animals we cannot be certain whether they are present in soil naturally or as a result of faecal contamination.

EXOGENOUS AND ENDOGENOUS INFECTION

When an individual suffers infection with organisms acquired from the sources mentioned above he is said to be infected from an *exogenous* source. Alternatively, *endogenous* infection may take place, i.e. the organism responsible for the disease has been living in or on the patient's tissues for some time. Reference has already been made (Chapter 4) to endogenous infection which can arise from essentially commensal species such as *Strept. viridans* or potentially pathogenic species which have been carried by the host for weeks or months before some alteration in the host-parasite relationship allows them to cause disease.

METHODS OF SPREAD OF INFECTION

More than 400 years ago Fracastorius's thesis *De contagione* detailed, in the first volume, his observations on the transmission of contagion from person to person; many of his ideas have been proved correct in the last few decades but we are still uncertain of the mechanisms involved in the spread of some infections.

Arthropod-borne blood infections
In such infections the causal microorganisms are present in the host's blood stream and are transmitted to a new host by blood-sucking arthropods such as mosquitoes, fleas, lice and ticks. In almost all such infections the microorganism can be spread only by its arthropod vector, but in certain cases the disease may affect tissues which allow transmission by other mechanisms, e.g. infection with bubonic plague is arthropod-borne to man from rats but occasional cases of plague also have a focus of infection in the lungs. Cases of pneumonic plague excrete the plague bacilli from their respiratory tract in large numbers so that the sputum of such cases is highly infectious to other men.

Venereal infections

The causative organisms of syphilis and gonorrhoea have very feeble powers of survival outside the human body, hence they must be transmitted speedily from host to host and in adult infection this is by sexual intercourse; there are of course, occasional instances of doctors and nurses being infected by careless examination of a syphilitic patient. Similarly, if the primary syphilitic lesion occurs on the lips or tongue of an individual who acquired the infection by abnormal sexual practices the causal organism can be transmitted to another person by kissing. Gonococcal infection of the eyes of babies can take place during birth if the mother is suffering from sexually acquired gonorrhoea. Similarly, occasional cases of gonococcal ophthalmia and vulvo-vaginitis can occur in young children infected from an adult attendant via sponges or damp towels.

Respiratory tract infections

In contrast with the spread of the above infections, a variety of methods of transmission occur in respiratory infections.

Organisms are expelled from cases of respiratory tract infection and by carriers of pathogenic species by spitting, nose-blowing and by their fingers; additionally they are disseminated by sneezing, laughing and coughing. Thus handkerchiefs, floors, furniture, clothing and other fabrics become contaminated with such secretions and these fomites can then act as vehicles of infection. Bacteria thus expelled can survive in the dust on surfaces for days or weeks and in the case of some pathogens even for months, e.g. tubercle bacilli, provided they are not exposed to direct sunlight.

Respiratory pathogens can thus be acquired in several ways, by *direct contact*, e.g. kissing, hand-shaking or by *indirect contact* where the new host transfers bacteria from clothing and other fomites with his hands into his nose or mouth.

Similarly *dust-borne* spread may occur when infected dust is made air-borne as when clothing is brushed or beds are made. Infected dust particles thus released may remain in the air for some time and be inhaled by the new host.

Finally, in addition to contact and dust-borne spread, a third method is possible namely, by *droplet spray*. Droplets of varying size are sprayed into the environment when we sneeze, cough, etc.; large droplets ($>0 \cdot 1$ mm in diameter) immediately fall on to surfaces and contribute to infected dust. *Small droplets* ($<0 \cdot 1$ mm in diameter) evaporate rapidly to form droplet-nuclei and because of their very small size

($<10\mu$m) remain air-borne and can be inhaled; in spite of the fact that droplet nuclei greatly outnumber large droplets they rarely contain bacteria and only in some virus infections are they thought to play a part in transmitting pathogenic organisms.

Surface infections

Infection of skin, wounds and burns are acquired by mechanisms similar to those operating in the transmission of respiratory tract pathogens.

Alimentary tract infections

As with the spread of respiratory tract infections there are several methods of transmitting organisms causing bowel infection. Bowel pathogens are excreted in the faeces of cases and carriers and are, in general, less resistant to environmental agents than those causing respiratory tract infections although many survive for several weeks provided they are in moist surroundings.

Water-borne spread of infection occurs if an untreated water supply is fouled with excreta of cases or carriers of infection; this method of spread is classically associated with typhoid fever and cholera. The fouled water need not necessarily be imbibed since infection may be acquired from its use in preparing salads and other foods.

Hand-borne infection is the principle method of spread in bacillary dysentery, particularly in well-developed communities with a safe water supply and methods of sewage disposal which prevent access of 'filthy, faecal-feeding flies' and other vectors to human excreta. A case or carrier will contaminate his hands while cleansing himself after de-faecation (filthy, faecal fingers) and the pathogens can be transferred to toilet chains, wash-basin taps, door handles etc., thence to the fingers of another person and from there into his mouth. Similarly, hospital personnel may contaminate their fingers from bed-pans, soiled linen etc., and in addition to the risk of infecting themselves they may contaminate other fomites, e.g. drinking carafes, and thus transmit infection to patients.

Food-borne spread takes place when an infected individual is involved in food preparation or in other culinary activities where he may contaminate pots or pans in which the food is being processed. If foodstuffs are not protected from rodents and insects these, too, contribute to its contamination and subsequent infection by ingestion.

Finally laboratory acquired infection, either from pathological material or laboratory cultures, is a risk not only for the professional laboratory staff but to students in training. When screw-capped containers are opened aerosols are released and may be inhaled; fingers become contaminated from cultures and from working surfaces and transfer bacteria to the mouth; accidental self-injection with needle and syringe is not unknown, and obvious precautions must be constantly in force. It is essential that certain manoeuvres are carried out in specially constructed and ventilated protective cabinets; eating and smoking must be forbidden in the laboratory.

THE COMPROMISED HOST

Many patients are rendered liable to infection, endogenous or exogenous in origin, by virtue of some predisposing lesion or other alteration in their physiological state or environment.

People may be compromised *extrinsically* and a few examples are:

(1) Admission to the hospital environment with the immediate and continuous bombardment by a battery of new microorganisms such as 'the hospital staphylococcus' and *Pseudomonas pyocyanea*.

(2) The use *and* abuse of antimicrobial agents with the attendant risk of alterations in their microbial flora which may be of potentially lethal significance, e.g. the onset of generalized candidosis.

(3) The need for aggressive therapy for neoplasia frequently requiring immunosuppressive procedures, e.g. in leukaemia and transplantation surgery which *pari passu* reduces the body defences against infection including infection with microorganisms which are essentially commensal in the healthy individual.

(4) Lack of isolation facilities. Isolation of an infected individual aims at reducing the risk of transmission of pathogens to other people (Source Isolation) or alternatively the isolation of patients known to be unusually susceptible to infection (Protective Isolation).

Similarly many people are *compromised intrinsically*, i.e. because of their physical state they are more likely to suffer infection than their healthy biological equivalent and examples of such intrinsic compromise are:

(1) The newborn
(2) The elderly
(3) Diabetics
(4) Cancer patients
(5) Candidates for transplant surgery
(6) Open-heart surgery

(7)   Those requiring hip replacement

(8)   Those seriously injured, burned or 'ill'

It is obvious that many intrinsically compromised patients must be subjected to extrinsic compromise and indeed it is surprising that any such individuals escape infection.

In patients compromised for one or more reasons endogenous infection is a real risk but we have available methods of reducing that risk; one example is the patient with a congenital or acquired heart defect which predisposes to subacute bacterial endocarditis. Such individuals must be kept in a good state of dental health and when they require dental treatment, whether of a conservative or radical nature, they should be screened bacteriologically to assess their buccal flora so that suitable peroperative antibiotic prophylaxis can be assured.

Likewise the risk of clostridial myonecrosis (gas gangrene) can be virtually eliminated in patients requiring amputation of the lower limb or hip replacement by peroperative penicillin prophylaxis; such preventive measures combined with pre-operative povidone-iodine soaks deal competently with *Cl. welchii* spores which inhabit the buttocks and surrounding skin and ensure the killing of any vegetative cells which may be in the operation area.

These two proven examples of prophylactic excellence are not always followed in clinical practice!

Neutropenia is a 'natural' state of compromise whether congenital or cyclic in origin but is more commonly seen in an iatrogenic situation, e.g. in patients being treated with cytotoxic agents as in acute leukaemia; whilst a granulocyte transfusion may be of *therapeutic* value we should endeavour to protect such individuals from unnecessary acquisition of hospital microorganisms by isolation and by monitoring their bacterial flora frequently so that impending opportunist pathogens can be recognized early and our therapeutic potential assessed before they attack.

It must be appreciated that infection in immunosuppressed patients rarely presents in typical fashion; this latter fact is known to nursing staff who are in constant attendance but is a lesson of which their medical colleagues are less appreciative.

INFLUENCE OF ANTIBIOTICS

Until the 1960s, Gram-positive cocci, and particularly *Staph. aureus*, dominated infections in compromised patients but the field is now led by Gram-negative aerobic bacilli particularly in patients on cytotoxic therapy.

This change in infecting species with *Ps. pyocyanea*, *Esch. coli* and Klebsiella species leading the league table is, at least in part, explained by such bacteria being more resistant to commonly used antibiotics and hospital disinfectants, their greater resistance to therapeutic cytotoxic agents and perhaps that immunosuppression (natural or therapeutically induced) selectively reduces the immune response to Gram-negative bacteria.

Reference has already been made to the value of the prophylactic use of antimicrobial agents in reducing the incidence of subacute bacterial endocarditis and also clostridial myonecrosis. On the other hand there are few proven instances of the prophylactic use of antibiotics in clinical practice; the most recent of these however serves to underline at least two facts, firstly, the need for controlled clinical trials to prove that antimicrobial agents may have a prophylactic merit and secondly that wherever possible the antimicrobial agent should have a *narrow* and if possible specific action. This double goal has been achieved in reports of the dramatic reduction of Bacteroides infection in colonic surgery with the peroperative administration of metronidazole (Flagyl). Even in this specific example it should be realized that the prophylactic use of antimicrobial agents must still be secondary to good surgical technique.

CHAPTER 12
Classification of bacteria

Bacteria are primarily subdivided into *lower* and *higher* groups. *Lower bacteria* (Eubacteria) are unicellular and each cell is biologically independent; they never occur as sheathed filaments and are much more numerous than higher bacteria. Almost all bacteria which are pathogenic to man and animals belong to the lower group.

By contrast, *higher bacteria* (Actinomycetales) are filamentous: some are sheathed and exhibit true branching with the formation of a mycelium; certain cells may have specialized functions, e.g. for reproduction, hence some interdependence occurs among higher bacteria. Only a very few are pathogenic to man; several useful antibiotics have been derived from higher bacteria, e.g. *Streptomyces griseus* produces streptomycin.

Lower bacteria are classified by their morphology and reactions to Gram's staining technique thus:

Cocci are globose cells, *Bacilli* appear as relatively straight cylindrical cells, *Vibrios* are definitely curved rod-shaped cells, *Spirilla* are spiralled non-flexous rods and *Spirochaetes* are very thin, spirally twisted flexous filaments (Fig. 10).

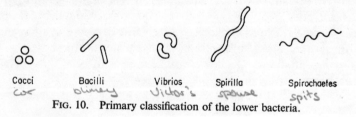

| Cocci | Bacilli | Vibrios | Spirilla | Spirochaetes |

FIG. 10.   Primary classification of the lower bacteria.

Each of these morphological kinds of lower bacteria are further subdivided on the basis of staining reactions or more detailed investigations.

70

COCCI +∪E GRAM (ECEPT
Neisseriae

Six main groups of cocci can be distinguished by noting their Gram staining reaction and the spatial relationship of cells, one to another, in each group. The groups correspond with biological genera and with the exception of one group, *Neisseriae*, all are Gram-positive (Fig. 11).

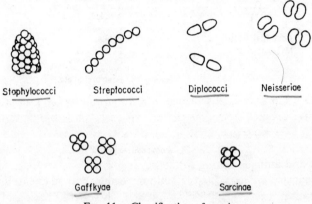

Staphylococci   Streptococci   Diplococci   Neisseriae

Gaffkyae   Sarcinae

FIG. 11. Classification of cocci.

grapes

Staphylococci occur as irregular clusters of cocci, lacking any orderly arrangement since successive cell divisions occur irregularly in different planes. chain

Streptococci adhere mainly in chains since consecutive planes of cleavage occur in the same axis.

Diplococci divide in a similar way to streptococci but adhere mainly in pairs and the cells in each pair are slightly elongate in the long axis of the pair. On *in-vitro* cultivation the cells become globose.

Neisseriae are Gram-negative; the cells adhere mainly in pairs and when seen in films of pathological material or from first cultures in the laboratory they are slightly elongate at right-angles to the axis of the pair.

Gaffkyae: division occurs consecutively in two planes at right-angles and hence they are seen as tetrads, i.e. flat plates of four cells.

Sarcinae are seen as cubes or packets of eight cells since division occurs consecutively in three planes at right-angles.

puro sarcina
are sporing

BACILLI

The primary subdivision of bacilli into groups is less exact than that for cocci and several of the groups described contain many biological

genera which can be differentiated only by detailed study of their biochemical, serological and other properties (Fig. 12).

Acid-fast bacilli, i.e. members of the genus *Mycobacterium*, are separable from other bacilli by virtue of their ability, once stained, to tolerate
attempted decolourization with strong mineral acids.

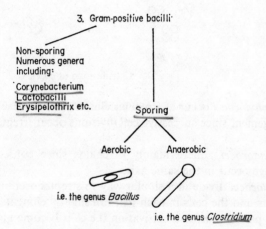

FIG. 12.   Classification of bacilli.

Bacilli which are not acid-fast can be classified into those which are
Gram-negative and others which are Gram-positive. Biological genera
within the Gram-negative group include *Pseudomonas*, *Salmonella*,
Shigella, *Escherichia*, *Proteus*, *Pasteurella*, *Brucella*, *Haemophilus* etc.

The Gram-positive group of bacilli may be subdivided into those
genera which form spores, i.e. the genus *Bacillus* whose members are
aerobic and the genus *Clostridium* whose members are anaerobic as well
as numerous genera which cannot form spores, e.g. *Corynebacterium*,
Lactobacillus, *Erysipelothrix* and *Listeria*.

Recognition of genera within the non-sporing Gram-positive bacilli and within Gram-negative bacilli demands more detailed study of morphological and other physiological attributes.

VIBRIOS AND SPIRILLA GRAM -VE

Vibrios, definitely curved rod-shaped cells, and Spirilla, non-flexuous spiralled rods, are Gram-negative; species can be recognized only by detailed cultural, biochemical and serological methods.

PATHOGENIC SPIROCHAETES -VE

These slim, spiralled, flexuous filaments are classified into three genera. Members of the genus *Borrelia* are larger than those of the other two genera and can be seen by the light microscope and are Gram-negative; they also have a larger coil wave-length (2–3 μm) and greater coil amplitude than the other genera (Fig. 13).

spirochaetes { Borrelia / Treponema \ Leptospira

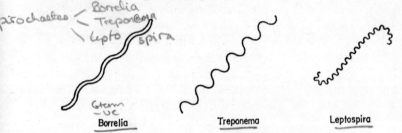

Gram -ve
Borrelia   **Treponema**   **Leptospira**

FIG. 13. Classification of spirochaetes.

Treponemata are much finer with a shorter coil wave-length (1 μm) of small amplitude; coils are more numerous than *Borrelia* and can be seen only by dark-ground microscopy or with the light microscope after staining by a silver impregnation technique.

Leptospirae are even finer than *Treponemata* and the coils are so close —wave-length of 0·5 μm—that they can hardly be seen under dark-ground microscopy. One or both ends of the organism are often recurved on the body.

ACTINOMYCETALES +VE

There are two genera of medical importance in the high bacteria.

Actinomyces are Gram-positive and mycelium-forming, usually also showing bacillary and coccal forms due to fragmentation and are anaerobic. The species infecting man grow in the tissues as colonies which become macroscopically visible.

Nocardia have many features in common with *Actinomyces* but they are aerobic and usually acid-fast.

Gram +ve = Cocci (except Neisseria) Bacillus — sporing
                actinomyces   corynebacterium

Gram −ve = Neisseria, Bacillus = E Coli shigella
              etc. Borrelia, Vibrios + Spirilla
Acid fast = mycobacterium + Nocardia

CHAPTER 13
Gram-positive cocci

STAPHYLOCOCCI

Morphology

Each cell is approximately 1μm in diameter and spherical; they occur in irregular clusters of varying size and when grown in fluid medium clustering may be less obvious and chain-formation may be seen. Usually non-capsulate but small capsules are detectable on freshly isolated pathogenic strains. Non-motile, non-sporing.

Cultural requirements

Grow over wide temperature range, 10–42°C. Optimum = 37°C. Aerobic and facultatively anaerobic and grow on the simplest of media.

Cultural appearances

Opaque, convex disks—2–4 mm after 24 hours incubation at 37°C, and pigmented. *Staph. aureus* = golden yellow, *Staph. albus* = white, *Staph. citreus* = lemon. Pigment formation is accentuated by growing on cream-agar.

Biochemical activities

Earlier methods of differentiating pathogenic from commensal staphylococci, e.g. fermentation of carbohydrates and ability to liquefy gelatin, have been superseded by the much more reliable *coagulase test*.

— *Coagulase Test*. Virtually all strains isolated from pathological material produce the enzyme coagulase whereas commensal strains rarely do so.

Five drops of an overnight broth culture of the strain to be tested are added to a tube containing 0·5 ml of a 1 in 10 dilution of citrated rabbit plasma, the diluent being sterile physiological saline. This tube and another inoculated with a known coagulase-producing strain are then

75

incubated at 37°C and inspected hourly; clotting of the plasma occurs, usually within 4–6 hr if the strain produces coagulase. A negative control tube, i.e. one containing diluted citrated plasma to which is added 5 drops of sterile physiological saline, should be included with each batch of tests to ensure that the plasma does not undergo auto-coagulation.

Phosphatase test. An alternative test of pathogenicity relies on the production of phosphatase by pathogenic strains of staphylococci; such activity is detected when strains are grown on plates containing phenol-phthalein phosphate. Phosphatase production is readily recognized by exposing the resultant growth to ammonia fumes when the liberation of phenolphthalein is revealed by phosphatase-producing colonies turning a bright pink colour.

In practice, the phosphatase test is normally restricted to the survey of nasal and perineal swab material from potential carriers.

Serological characteristics
Strains can be typed using agglutination techniques with absorbed antisera but serological typing has been replaced by phage-typing which is more sensitive and more reliable.

Phage-typing. Phages are viruses which show a high degree of specificity for their host bacteria and produce lysis of the host cell. Thus if a plate of suitable medium is sown with a lawn of susceptible coagulase-positive staphylococci and suitable phage-preparations are individually applied, then after incubation there will be, at the site of implantation of certain phages, an absence of bacterial growth indicating that the particular phage was capable of lysing the staphylococci. By noting the pattern of growth-inhibition we can identify the phage-type of the staphylococcus.

Epidemiology of staphylococcal infections
Infections caused by staphylococci range from simple skin lesions, e.g. a furuncle, to more deep-seated conditions such as acute osteomyelitis. Sometimes there is an extension from the primary lesion which results in septicaemia or pyaemia with abscess formation in many organs and tissues.

The sources of *Staph. aureus* are other individuals who are either carriers or are suffering from infection; *endogenous* infection may occur in a person carrying the same phage-type in his anterior nares or perineum as that isolated from his lesion.

A carrier or case of infection will disseminate staphylococci into the

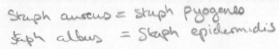

environment from his clothing, skin squames and lesion and a susceptible host may become infected indirectly from fomites in the environment or directly by contact with the case or carrier. Such *exogenous* infection is the rule in hospital-acquired staphylococcal infection which usually involves wounds although staphylococcal pneumonia may also result.

Certain staphylococci produce enterotoxins which, unlike other staphylococcal toxins, are heat-stable and can even survive boiling for short periods. If enterotoxin-producing staphyloccocci contaminate foodstuffs on which they can survive or grow, anyone ingesting such materials may suffer acute, toxic-type, food poisoning.

On rare occasions animals may be the source of infection.

Prevention

It will be obvious that exogenous infection in hospital could be controlled to a large extent if susceptible individuals were separated from carriers and cases of staphylococcal infection. Except in a few instances, such as patients being prepared for transplantation surgery, it is impossible in existing hospitals to ensure that sources of infection and susceptibles do not meet or share the same environment.

However, *contamination of the environment* can be reduced if intelligent measures are undertaken. For example, lesions must be covered with an impervious material and they should be dressed only in a dressings station and *not* in the open ward; wherever possible infected individuals should be nursed in isolation; carriage should be suppressed by applying suitable antimicrobial creams; and a continuing awareness of the part played by hands in spreading the organism from person to person should dictate a high level of personal hygiene. *Control of organisms in the environment* can be effected by oiling of floors, bedclothes, towels, pyjamas, etc. so that infected dust and other materials are trapped on the surface and are incapable of redissemination. Wet vacuuming of impervious floor surfaces is ideal but if the structure does not allow such treatment damp sweeping and dusting should be undertaken. Operating and dressings rooms should be properly ventilated with a positive pressure system so that air enters from outside the hospital and is not sucked in from corridors and wards.

Viability

Thermal death point (TDP) = $62°C/\frac{1}{2}$ hr. Survives outside the host more readily and longer than most other non-sporing bacteria; if protected from direct sunlight strains can exist in dust, bed-clothing, curtains, etc. for weeks or months.

Susceptible to disinfectants if these are used at correct concentrations.

STREPTOCOCCI

Morphology

Approximately 1μm in diameter, spherical and occurring usually in chains of varying length; when grown on solid medium some degree of clustering may be noted. Capsules occur in certain types when freshly isolated. Non-motile, non-sporing.

Cultural requirements

Similar to staphylococci but grow better on enriched medium, e.g. blood agar; narrower temperature range, i.e. 22–42°C.

Cultural appearances

Circular, low convex disks, semi-transparent and 0·5–1 mm in diameter after 24 hr incubation at 37°C; their small diameter and the absence of pigmentation allow ready differentiation from staphylococcal colonies. Three types of response may be noted when streptococci are grown on blood agar but the colonies themselves are identical regardless of change in the medium.

α-Haemolytic streptococci are surrounded by a narrow halo of greenish discolouration of the blood agar medium; lysis of the red cells does not occur.

β-Haemolytic strains produce a much wider zone of complete haemolysis.

γ-Haemolytic (non-haemolytic) streptococci produce no alteration in the medium.

Since these three cultural types of streptococci differ in other biological characteristics and also in their clinical manifestations they require separate description.

α-HAEMOLYTIC STREPTOCOCCI (*STREPT. VIRIDANS*)

Biochemical activities

Although there have been many attempts to differentiate species within the group no practical classification has emerged. In identification, the most important point is differentiation from pneumococci which may appear very similar on cultivation on blood agar. This is most readily performed by testing for bile solubility or sensitivity to 'optochin' since *Strept. viridans* react negatively whereas pneumococci (q.v.) give positive reactions.

Serological characteristics

The fact that viridans streptococci are essentially commensal and do not spread epidemically may explain the relative lack of interest in their antigenic structure; thus what little is known, e.g. that they do not possess C-group antigens like β-haemolytic streptococci, is entirely academic.

Infections caused by *Strept. viridans*

These are always endogenous; such organisms are frequently found in carious teeth and are commonly present in periapical infections; otherwise they lead an essentially commensal existence in the buccal cavity of all persons. However, *Strept. viridans* is the most common cause of subacute bacterial endocarditis; this infection, which was invariably fatal before the introduction of antibiotics, occurs in individuals with predisposing cardiac lesions which may be *congenital*, e.g. patent ductus arteriosus, or *acquired*, e.g. rheumatic endocarditis. Such people are particularly at risk if they are in a poor state of dental hygiene when, even during normal mastication and more so during dental therapy, large showers of *Strept. viridans* enter the blood stream and may settle on the damaged heart valves or other areas.

Prevention

Individuals with heart lesions known to carry a risk of developing subacute bacterial endocarditis should be kept in an excellent state of dental hygiene and additionally must be given suitable antibiotic cover, during and for 48 hr after having dental treatment even of a minor nature.

β-HAEMOLYTIC STREPTOCOCCI

Biochemical activities

None of any practical use for purposes of identification.

Serological characteristics

Since these streptococci are the most common in infections of man and many animals, they have been subjected to rigorous antigenic analysis and the results have great importance in epidemiological practice. They are broadly subdivided into *serogroups* by testing for the presence of a particular group-specific carbohydrate antigen present in the cell wall. This carbohydrate or C-antigen can be extracted from the cell wall and its identity established by precipitation tests against group-specific antisera. Thus 15 serological groups A–Q (none designated I or J) can be recognized and group-A strains account for almost all human β-haemolytic streptococcal infections—such strains are named *Strept. pyogenes.*

Strept. pyogenes can be further classified into highly specific *serotypes* in precipitation tests with type-specific antisera prepared against their M-antigens. Each M-antigen is specific for its serotype strains, is protein in nature and is located at or near the cell surface. The M-antigens are also directly related to the pathogenicity of *Strept. pyogenes* since M-antibodies protect against infection with the homologous serotype; and strains which have lost the ability to produce M-antigen are non-pathogenic.

Thus *Strept. pyogenes* strains isolated from individuals involved in an epidemic situation can be serotyped and the source of the epidemic traced and removed.

A recent useful addition to typing procedures is afforded by serologically specific opacity factors (O.F.); O.F. production is confined to certain members of certain serotypes of Group A streptococci and can be readily recognized by tube or slide testing. In the slide test for O.F. a glass slide is coated with agar to which has been added horse serum; spot inoculation of either a culture supernate of the organism or acid extract is made and the slide incubated in a moist chamber at 37°C overnight.

Opacity is obvious at those sites inoculated with O.F. producing strains; type specific inhibition of the opacity reaction can be demonstrated by incorporating active O.F. supernate with the agar and horse serum and when anti O.F. serum is placed on the surface clear areas of inhibition are seen when the anti O.F. serum is specific for the incorporated O.F. supernate.

Epidemiology of *Strept. pyogenes* infections

Strept. pyogenes is very commonly the cause of tonsillitis and pharyngitis; quinsy throat (tonsillar abscess) occurs as a complication. In individuals infected with strains which produce erythrogenic toxin and who do not possess immunity to the latter a characteristic punctate erythematous skin rash develops and they are then said to be suffering from scarlet fever. It must be emphasized that cases of scarlet fever are no more, and certainly no less, dangerous as a source of infection to others than cases of infection without the skin rash. *Strept. pyogenes* also causes other syndromes and frequently displays its ability to spread locally to adjacent tissues—e.g. adenitis, mastoiditis and otitis media may occur as complications of tonsillitis; it is also the cause of erysipelas and some cases of impetigo and occurs in wounds, burns and, until recently, was the commonest cause of puerperal sepsis.

Sources of infection are cases suffering from any one of the various syndromes produced by such organisms and carriers who most commonly are throat carriers; however, nasal carriage, although much less common, is more dangerous to susceptible individuals since it has been demonstrated that nasal carriers account for as many fresh infections in other individuals as do throat carriers. As with staphylococcal infections, cases and carriers of *Strept. pyogenes* extensively contaminate their clothing and the general environment and other people may become infected by direct contact, or indirectly via fomites. Airborne spread by dust particles or rarely by droplet spray also plays a part in spreading such organisms.

Acute rheumatism

The causal role of *Strept. pyogenes* in acute rheumatic fever and other non-pyogenic sequelae of infection is now beyond doubt, although the mechanism whereby the organism produces the non-septic rheumatic complications some 2–3 weeks after the initial infection is still a source of debate and research. There is no association with any particular serotype and the risk of acute rheumatism, but certain subsidiary factors predispose, e.g. social circumstances, including poor nutrition, and geographic factors. It is usually stated that rheumatic fever and carditis are more common in temperate zones but this is not so and many cases occur in tropical countries. It would appear that altitude is an important determining factor since it is known that the primary streptococcal infection causing rheumatic fever becomes less common with increasing altitude.

Acute glomerulonephritis

This also occurs as a non-suppurative complication of *Strept. pyogenes* infection. In contrast with rheumatic sequelae glomerulonephritis is associated only with infections caused by very few serotypes with type-12 strains predominating; not all type-12 strains are nephrotoxic and other serotypes of which some strains may be nephrotoxic belong to types 4 and 25.

Prevention
Occasionally group-A streptococcal infection is endogenous in origin, particularly in erysipelas, but the majority of infections caused by *Strept. pyogenes* are acquired exogenously and prophylactic measures are the same as those for staphylococcal infection.

However, we have a most valuable means of preventing the spread of infection by *Strept. pyogenes*, i.e. the prompt and adequate treatment of cases with penicillin; this is possible since such organisms have remained eminently sensitive to this antibiotic and have not acquired the resistance which is so obvious in staphylococci, particularly in hospital strains of the latter.

Similarly, adequate treatment of streptococcal sore throat and other lesions with penicillin eliminates the risk of acute rheumatism and individuals who have a previous history of acute rheumatism should be protected against further streptococcal infection by continuous penicillin prophylaxis.

Unhappily penicillin treatment of streptococcal infection by nephrotoxic strains is not so efficient in protecting against acute glomerulonephritis. Even with early administration of penicillin in doses adequate to eliminate the causal organism one can expect little more than a 50% reduction in the incidence of acute nephritis.

Group B strains of β-haemolytic streptococci
The significance of such strains in causing infection in the puerperium and in the neonate is being recognized. Since Group B strains are commensal in the alimentary tract and also inhabit the vulva and vagina of a proportion of women, they probably act as opportunist pathogens. The majority of Group B strains can be readily recognized by their distinctive colonial appearance when grown on Columbia agar under anaerobic conditions.

γ-HAEMOLYTIC STREPTOCOCCI (*STREPT. FAECALIS, ENTEROCOCCI*)

Strains are usually oval in shape and occur in short chains. Unlike α- and β-haemolytic strains, *Enterococci* can grow on media containing bile salts, e.g. MacConkey's, and the colonies are minute, 0·5 mm in diameter, and usually magenta-coloured.

Biochemical activities
In addition to their ability to grow on bile salt media, *Enterococci* can also grow in the presence of 6·5% NaCl and ferment mannitol with

gas-production, properties not shared by other streptococci. Four biochemical types, one of which occurs as three variants, may be recognized on the basis of gelatin liquefaction, fermentation of sorbitol and arabinose and other features.

Serological characteristics
All strains possess a C-antigen and belong to serogroup D.

Infections caused by Enterococci
Enterococci are essentially commensal in the intestine but can give rise to endogenous urinary tract infections, usually in association with Gram-negative bowel bacilli but occasionally as the sole cause.

Viability of Streptococci
It has already been noted that the temperature range over which streptococci will grow is narrower than that of staphylococci, their TDP is also lower, i.e. 54°C/½ hr, except that *Strept. faecalis* again is exceptional and has a TDP of 60°C/½ hr. The survival of streptococci outside the host is similar to that of staphylococci. *Strept pyogenes* is very much more resistant to crystal violet than are staphylococci and this fact allows us to make a blood agar plate selective for isolating *Strept. pyogenes* by incorporating a concentration of 1 in 500 000 crystal violet in the medium. Staphylococci on throat swabs will not tolerate such a concentration whereas *Strept. pyogenes* flourish.

PNEUMOCOCCI (DIPLOCOCCUS PNEUMONIAE: STREPT. PNEUMONIAE)

Morphology
Each cell is approximately 1 μm in its long axis, slightly elongated (lanceolate) and cells adhere in pairs with their long axes in 'line-ahead formation'; short chains are also noted. Non-motile, non-sporing; capsules of varying size can be seen on strains freshly isolated from pathological material but capsulation diminishes and is eventually lost on continued *in vitro* cultivation. Similarly, laboratory cultures lose their lanceolate shape and become spherical after one or two subcultures.

Cultural requirements
Temperature range is even more restricted than streptococci—25–40°C. Growth is enhanced if cultivation takes place in an atmosphere of 5% CO_2 and similarly the addition of 0·1% glucose to the medium is beneficial.

Recent evidence confirms that unless anaerobic conditions (i.e. an atmosphere of 90% hydrogen and 10% carbon dioxide) are used for attempted isolation, less than 50% of pneumococci will be recovered.

Cultural appearances
Colonies are similar in size to those of streptococci and are surrounded by a zone of α-haemolysis so that they may be confused with *Strept. viridans*, although pneumococcal colonies are plateau-shaped and not convex and ultimately the colonies develop an elevated edge and concentric ridges—the draughtsman colony.

Biochemical activities
Interest in these is restricted to tests which allow differentiation from *Strept. viridans*. Earlier tests have been superseded by determining the 'optochin' sensitivity of the isolate; pneumococci are extremely sensitive and viridans streptococci are resistant to 'optochin'. The test is performed by sowing the strain under test on a blood agar plate and then placing a filter paper disk, impregnated with a 1 in 4000 aqueous solution of 'optochin' on the surface of the medium. Incubation for 18 hr at 37°C will reveal a zone of inhibition of growth surrounding the disk if the isolate is a pneumococcus, whereas *Strept. viridans* will grow right up to the disk margin.

Another test which is equally reliable but technically tiresome is the bile solubility test; pneumococci are soluble in bile whereas *Strept. viridans* is not. One part of a sterile 10% solution of sodium taurocholate in normal soline is added to 10 parts of a broth culture of the organism under test and the mixture is then incubated at 37°C for 15 min. Lysis of the pneumococci is revealed by a clearing of the originally turbid mixture. The bile salt solution used must be crystal clear and the pH of the broth culture must be checked and if necessary adjusted to between 7 and 7·5, otherwise acid precipitation of the bile salt will result in turbidity.

Serological characteristics
Serotyping of pneumococci is dependent on the highly specific capsular polysaccharides against which specific antisera can be produced for typing purposes. There are more than 75 serotypes of pneumococci. When a suspension of pneumococci is mixed with specific antiserum on a microscope slide and the preparation is viewed through an oil-immersion objective the capsules are sharply demarcated and appear swollen, whereas if mixed with heterologous antiserum the capsule is not visible.

The use of the term 'capsule-swelling reaction' for the test is quite misleading since there is no increase in the size of the capsule which merely becomes obvious because of precipitation occurring between the capsular antigen and its specific antibody.

Epidemiology of pneumococcal infections

Lobar pneumonia is the disease which we primarily associate with pneumococci but they are also frequently involved as secondary pathogens in cases of bronchopneumonia where the primary infection is caused by a virus, e.g. in measles or influenza. Pneumococci are incriminated in a proportion of cases of acute pyogenic meningitis, either as a complication of pneumonia or as a primary illness. Individuals with traumatic or congenital defects in the skull may suffer recurrent attacks of pneumococcal meningitis unless the defect is repaired surgically. Pneumococci are also implicated in some cases of otitis media and conjunctivitis. Sources of pneumococcal infection are cases and carriers, and most pneumococcal infections are exogenously acquired. The modes of spread are the same as those of other organisms excreted from the respiratory tract. However, when pneumococci are involved as secondary invaders in bronchopneumonia, serotyping studies show that they are almost always the same type as those inhabiting the patient's upper respiratory tract and the super-infection is endogenous.

Prevention

General prophylactic procedures are the same as those used in the case of streptococcal infections. There are certain circumstances where a high incidence of lobar pneumonia, caused by only a few epidemic serotypes, can justify the use of active immunization with a polyvalent capsular antigen; in controlled trials a satisfactory degree of protection was noted. However, one could not justify immunization in normal communities when pneumococcal pneumonia is sporadic, responds readily to antimicrobial drugs and is not economically significant.

Viability

Although the TDP of pneumococci is lower than that of other Gram-positive cocci (52°C/15 min) and is more difficult to maintain in the laboratory, it has reasonable powers of survival outside the human host. This is evidenced by the fact that it can be recovered from the dust in the crevices between wood flooring boards some weeks after a room has been inhabited by a case or carrier.

CHAPTER 14
Neisseriae

Morphology
All members of the genus *Neisseria* appear as oval diplococci, each cell measuring approximately 1μm in its largest diameter. The longer diameters of each pair are parallel—'line-abreast formation'—and the opposed surfaces are flattened or concave. Non-motile, non-sporing. The two pathogenic members of the genus *N. meningitidis* (the meningococcus) and *N. gonorrhoeae* (the gonococcus) become spherical on sub-cultivation; these pathogens are characteristically intracellular in films made from pathological material; capsules are visible if specific antiserum is applied to wet preparations of the material as submitted to the laboratory or of colonies of the first laboratory isolates. The ability to form capsules disappears rapidly on *in-vitro* cultivation.

Cultural requirements
The pathogenic species are most fastidious, the gonococcus even more so than the meningococcus since the former will grow only on media containing blood or serum; temperature ranges for growth emphasize the more demanding nature of the gonococcus (30–39°C) as compared with the meningococcus (25–42°C). The growth of each species is enhanced by cultivation in an atmosphere of 5% CO_2.

By contrast the various commensal members of the genus grow readily on ordinary media and over a wide range of temperature—even at room temperature!

Cultural appearances
There is considerable variation in colonial morphology but the pathogenic species usually appear as small semi-transparent disks after 24 hr at 37°C. Frequently on primary isolation the growth of gonococci may

be slow and not evident for two or more days. Commensal species produce more opaque colonies which are frequently larger than those of the pathogenic neisseriae although some, particularly those of *Neisseria flava*, may resemble closely those of meningococci.

Biochemical activities
All members of the genus give a positive oxidase reaction, i.e. colonies show a rapidly deepening purple colour when a freshly prepared 1% solution of tetramethyl-p-phenylene-diamine hydrochloride is applied to them. N.B. The re-agent is lethal to neisseriae if left in contact for more than 3–4 min, thus if colonies are to be subjected to further study they should be subcultured within the time limit stated.

Meningococci and gonococci can be readily differentiated from each other and from commensal neisseriae by performing fermentation tests using as substrates glucose, maltose and sucrose, but these must be contained in serum broth or agar and not peptone water so that the exacting pathogens will grow.

Meningococci ferment glucose and maltose only and gonococci only utilize glucose; commensal species either ferment all three substrates or alternatively do not attack any.

Serological characteristics
Meningococci belong to one of four groups, A–D and can be classified by agglutination tests with group-specific antisera. Gonococci have so far defied such exact antigenic characterization and seem to be serologically heterogenous.

Epidemiology of Neisserial infections
Commensal members of the genus live on mucous membranes including the buccal cavity, throat and urethra; they play no part in disease causation so far as we are aware.

Meningococcal infections
Meningococci are the most common cause of acute pyogenic meningitis which occurs sporadically and occasionally in epidemic form, particularly in military barracks or camps, or other establishments where a population is herded together in close proximity. Septicaemia, frequently running a chronic course and without meningeal involvement, is also associated with this organism and such cases may be labelled as pyrexias of uncertain origin until blood-culture is undertaken during an acute episode.

During epidemics of meningococcal meningitis serogroup-A strains predominate, whereas isolates from healthy carriers usually belong to groups B, C or D and it is thought that members of these groups are less pathogenic and/or less communicable.

The annually increasing incidence of meningococcal meningitis in Britain, starting in 1967, climbed to a peak in 1974; there were even fewer cases notified in 1976 than in 1975, although even in 1976 there were significantly more cases notified than in 1967. One hopes that this downward trend continues.

Viability
TDP of pathogenic members is 55°C/5 min or less and they are extremely susceptible to natural drying, sunlight and other invironmental features either natural or artificially produced by man. Hence they are obligate human parasites. The speed with which meningococci die when discharged from the respiratory tract demands that their spread from human cases or carriers is fairly intimate and is probably by direct contact, e.g. kissing or perhaps by the recipient host breathing in large infected droplets of saliva when a case or carrier sneezes or coughs in close proximity. The exact method of spread is still in doubt.

Prevention
Apart from isolation of cases and elimination of overcrowding during epidemics coupled with good natural ventilation, no specific methods are available.

Gonococcal infection
Gonorrhoea is a venereal infection spread by sexual intercourse and the feeble viability of the organism outside the host belies the occasional claim that infection was acquired from toilet seats. Gonococcal ophthalmia neonatorum may result during the birth of a baby if the mother is suffering from sexually acquired infection and occasional cases of infection, either conjunctivitis or vulvovaginitis, still occur in children's institutions and are transmitted from an infected adult with poor personal hygiene via communal sponges and towels.

It must be appreciated that although acute infection in the male is invariably accompanied by obvious symptoms, 50% or thereabouts of such infection in the female may be symptomless.

Recent reports of the isolation of β-lactamase producing strains of *N. gonorrhoeae* in several countries must raise anxieties regarding the value of penicillin therapy in the near future.

Prevention

Sexually acquired gonorrhoea is preventable by obvious methods; neonatal ophthalmia can be eliminated by ensuring that the mother is free from infection or alternatively by treating the potentially infected baby's eyes immediately after birth.

The other institutional types of non-sexually acquired infection can be prevented if nursing and medical attendants are free from infection or seek treatment and remain off duty until they are known to be cured.

CHAPTER 15
Acid-fast bacilli

MYCOBACTERIUM TUBERCULOSIS

Morphology
Straight or slightly curved rods, variable in size but approximately $3\mu m$
$\times 0\cdot3\mu m$; non-motile, non-capsulate, non-sporing; Gram-positive, but
difficult to stain by Gram's method; acid- **and** alcohol-fast. The five
types of tubercle bacilli cannot be differentiated on morphological
grounds.

Cultural requirements
Strict aerobes; the two types pathogenic for man, *Myco. tuberculosis*
(human type) and *Myco. bovis* (bovine type), have a fairly restricted
temperature range for growth, i.e. 30–41°C, and the optimum temperature is 37°C as is that of the murine type of bacillus. Avian tubercle
bacilli have a slightly higher optimum temperature, 43°C, and the
piscine or cold-blooded type grows best at 25°C. All types require a
rich medium, e.g. Lowenstein-Jensen's (L–J), and even then visible
growth does not appear for some *weeks*. Occasionally growth cannot
be detected until eight or more weeks have passed, even with incubation
under optimal conditions.

Further consideration is given only to the two types pathogenic for man
but it should be noted that the three other types can be differentiated
from each other and from human and bovine type bacilli by noting their
cultural appearance and more particularly by demonstrating their
differing virulence for various kinds of experimental animal.

Cultural appearances
On L–J glycerol-egg medium, *Myco. tuberculosis* produces a dry,
irregular, buff-coloured growth which is difficult to emulsify, whereas

the growth of bovine-type bacilli is moist, smooth white and readily suspended. The growth of the latter type on a glycerol-containing medium is less luxuriant than that of *Myco. tuberculosis*.

Biochemical activities
What little is known of these has no significance to the clinical bacteriologist.

Serological characters
Four main sero-groups of tubercle bacilli are recognized, but the human and bovine types are antigenically indistinguishable so that sero-identification is of no value in the clinical bacteriology laboratory.

Animal pathogenicity
Guinea-pigs are highly susceptible to human and bovine type bacilli and are used frequently in diagnostic laboratory practice; in areas where cases of human disease are discovered at a very early stage, guinea-pigs inoculated with sputum etc, may show infection where attempted *in vitro* cultivation of the bacilli on L–J medium fails. On occasion there may be difficulty in deciding whether a particular isolate is of the human or bovine type and such doubts can readily be resolved by injecting the stain subcutaneously into a rabbit—'the bovine goes for the bunny'— i.e. bovine-type tubercle bacilli cause progressive disease within a few weeks and at post-mortem miliary spread of the lesions is obvious. By contrast the human-type bacilli do not cause infection in the rabbit, or at the very most a local lesion may result.

Epidemiology of tuberculosis
Sources of infection are cases of pulmonary tuberculosis in other human beings and the new host is usually infected by breathing in bacilli lying in his environment. It is unlikely that droplet nuclei expelled by an infected individual contribute to the spread since the nuclei are too small to contain even one bacillus. Infection by inhalation usually results in pulmonary infection.

In communities where cattle suffer from infection with bovine-type bacilli and no attempt is made to eliminate these from the milk, man becomes infected by drinking the milk. Infection by ingestion most commonly causes intestinal tuberculosis.

It is worth noting that an upsurge in tubercle-infected cattle in south-west England in the last five years is directly associated with an increase of bovine-type infection in wild badgers; it is assumed that the latter contaminated pasture land thus acting as a sources of infection for the cattle.

However, both the human and bovine types have been incriminated regardless of the tissue or tract involved.

Primary tuberculosis in the lung usually gives rise to a small sub-pleural lesion with associated caseation ot the hilar lymph glands. This pathological picture is known as the Ghon focus and almost invariably heals by fibrosis and calcification and the individual develops a positive tuberculin reaction. Post-primary tuberculosis may be endogenous since the bacilli which caused the Ghon focus can remain viable even in the healed, calcified lesion. As opposed to re-activation, post-primary tuberculosis may result from re-infection from another case. An important difference in the pathology of post-primary infection as compared with primary tuberculosis is that lymph gland involvement is less common in the former and the tissue lesions are progressive with cavitation; therefore the post-primary case is a greater danger to other people.

Prevention

The dramatic reduction in the incidence of human infection by *Myco. bovis* which has followed the control of bovine-type tuberculosis and pasteurization of milk underlines the importance of setting up and maintaining cattle herds which are free from infection.

Similarly, the use of BCG (Bacille Calmette-Guérin) vaccine to protect susceptible individuals has resulted in a significant reduction in the disease. In carefully controlled trials an 80% reduction in incidence was obtained and it was shown also that vaccination gave complete protection against the more serious types of infection, i.e. miliary tuberculosis and tuberculous meningitis. Another vaccine made from a murine strain, the vole vaccine, was also tested in these trials and was, at least, equally efficacious. Other prophylactic measures include the elimination of overcrowding and malnutrition which are known to increase the risk of infection; similarly regular radiographic examination, especially of those with an occupational risk, allows earlier diagnosis and hence more rapid cure. Tuberculosis is one of the few diseases where adequate disinfection, e.g. by formalin vapour, of rooms and furnishings, used by patients must be carried out before occupation by other people. A small but continuing resurgence of tuberculosis has been noted in recent years affecting particularly men of middle age and, disproportionately so, those of a professional status.

OTHER MYCOBACTERIA

(1) Intermediate group

Several types which, in so far as pathogenicity for the human host is concerned, are intermediate between tubercle bacilli and the saprophytic acid-fast mycobacteria have attracted attention within recent years. These are associated with chronic ulceration of the skin and in the case of one organism, *Mycobacterium balnei*, there is evidence that infection was acquired in swimming pools and entered through skin abrasions. *Mycobacterium ulcerans*, first described more than twenty years ago in Australia, produces essentially similar lesions. *Myco. balnei* and *Myco. ulcerans* can be differentiated from each other and from tubercle bacilli by various methods and in particular have optimum temperatures for growth between 30–33°C and grow poorly, if at all, at 37°—the optimum for tubercle bacilli.

(2) Anonymous group

Members of this group have been isolated alone and in pure cultures from cases of 'pulmonary tuberculosis' but are readily differentiated from human and bovine type bacilli. In many instances members of the anonymous group are undoubtedly responsible for the tissue lesions whereas in others they have acted as secondary invaders in a true tuberculous infection. Unlike tubercle bacilli all anonymous mycobacteria can form the enzyme arylsulphatase and they are subdivided into *photochromogens* (which produce pigment only when exposed to the light), *scotochromogens* (which can produce pigment even when growing in the dark) and non-chromogens (which occur as colourless colonies or have very slow pigment production on exposure to light). Various other biological properties allow detailed differentiation of strains.

(3) Saprophytic and commensal group

Numerous species can be recognized; they grow very rapidly and on ordinary media. The only members of the group with significance to the medical bacteriologist are firstly *Myco. smegmatis* which occurs commensally in the smegma of men and women and may therefore be present in specimens of urine submitted from suspect cases of genito-urinary tuberculosis. Its presence in such specimens need not cause confusion, since although it is acid-fast it is usually readily decolourized by alcohol. It is also less tolerant of the chemical methods used in concentrating specimens for cultivation and animal inoculation; even if it escapes the concentration technique its rapid growth on other media and lack of virulence for guinea-pigs allows ready differentiation from tubercle bacilli. Similarly saprophytic mycobacteria often inhabit water pipes and taps so that one should ensure that water used for preparing reagents for Z–N staining and for washing films during such staining is free from such species.

MYCOBACTERIUM LEPRAE

This organism is regarded as being the causative agent in human leprosy although the association is suspected solely on the fulfilment of the first of Koch's postulates. *Myco. leprae* has not been isolated and attempts at experimental reproduction of the disease by implanting lepromatous material from a case into animals have not resulted in established disease.

One therefore must rely, for diagnostic purposes, on the microscopic demonstration of acid-fast bacilli in material taken from a suspect lesion; the leprosy bacillus is not as acid-fast as the tubercle bacillus and the strength of sulphuric acid used in attempted decolourization should be 5% and not 20% as is used for demonstrating acid-fastness in tubercle bacilli.

The organism would appear to have a low infectivity and may spread by direct contact with a very long incubation period but we are still ignorant of the exact mechanism of spread; opinions vary as to the prophylactic value of BCG vaccination and controlled trials are being undertaken in Uganda and Burma.

CHAPTER 16
Aerobic Gram-positive bacilli

CORYNEBACTERIA

Several species are commensal in man and others are pathogenic for certain domestic animals but one member of the genus, *Corynebacterium diphtheriae*, is pathogenic to man and gives rise to diphtheria; another species, *C. ulcerans*, is incriminated in the sore throat syndrome.

C. DIPHTHERIAE

Morphology
Size and shape are variable, particularly in films made from colonies after laboratory isolation. Expansion of one pole to give a club-shaped organism is frequently seen. Incomplete separation of cell walls during division leads to 'Chinese-letter' arrangement. More easily decolourized in Gram's staining method than most other Gram-positive organisms. Volutin granules, demonstrable, e.g. by Albert's staining technique, appear in preparations made from colonies on rich media such as serum-agar and are scanty or absent in films of colonies from selective tellurite-containing media. Non-capsulate, non-motile, non-sporing.

Cultural requirements
Aerobic, wide temperature range for growth—20–40°C—optimum 37°C. Grows on ordinary media but best on media containing serum or blood.

Cultural appearances
On serum media, e.g. Loeffler's, growth is very rapid and after 12–18 hr at 37°C circular grey colonies can be noted; these have a regular edge

but the colonies increase in size after 24–48 hr incubation and the edges are then crenated. Volutin granules are abundant in films made from such media; since many other organisms will also grow in Loeffler's serum medium it is customary to inoculate a selective medium containing tellurite at the same time as the serum medium.

Tellurite media suppress the growth of most other organisms likely to be present in the throat-swab specimen and also are slightly inhibitory to *C. diphtheriae*. Incubation, therefore, should be continued for 48–72 hr if no growth is apparent at 24 hr.

Three colonial types of *C. diphtheriae* can be distinguished on tellurite media and these are termed *gravis*, *mitis*, and *intermedius* variants since respectively they are generally associated with severe, mild and moderate clinical illness; all types reduce the tellurite in the medium so that the colonies are grey or black. No detailed description of the colonies is offered since these vary and in any case recognition is a matter of practice and expertise. In general, *gravis* and *mitis* types are similar in size but the former often has an irregular crenated edge with radial striations, whereas *mitis* type colonies are usually convex and circular in outline. *Intermedius* types produce colonies which are smaller in size and frequently have a flattened border which is circular; colonies of this type are black as opposed to the slate-grey colour of the other types. The few organisms other than diphtheria bacilli which grow on tellurite media can, by the expert, be differentiated from them on colonial appearance.

Biochemical activities
All the colonial types ferment glucose but only *gravis* strains ferment glycogen; they can be further differentiated by noting their varying haemolytic activities against ox and rabbit red cells and in tube haemolysis tests *gravis* strains lyse only rabbit cells, *intermedius* strains have no effect on either type of red cell whereas *mitis* strains lyse both ox and rabbit cells.

Serological characteristics
The three bio-types of *C. diphtheriae* are readily separable by antigenic analysis and each can also be subdivided by tests with agglutinating antisera. Diphtheria bacilli produce a powerful exotoxin which spreads throughout the patient's body and causes general toxaemia with obvious clinical effects on the circulatory and nervous systems and on renal tissues. The few strains of each bio-type which are non-toxigenic cannot cause diphtheria.

Animal pathogenicity

Several laboratory animals are susceptible to diphtheria exotoxin but usually guinea-pigs are used to determine whether an isolate is toxigenic. Two guinea-pigs are used in toxigenicity testing and one animal, protected by intraperitoneal administration of diphtheria antitoxin, acts as a control. Both control and test guinea-pigs have their abdomens shaved before 0·2 ml of a 12 hr culture of the isolate is injected intradermally. Toxigenic, i.e. virulent bacilli will produce a local erythematous area which within 32–48 hr will become necrotic, but in the control animal no reaction will occur. If neither animal shows a reaction the strain is non-toxigenic and if both animals react then the organism is not a diphtheria bacillus. Toxigenicity can also be determined *in vitro* by a gel-diffusion technique.

Epidemiology of diphtheria

Sources of infection are cases of the disease and carriers of virulent bacilli; both nose and throat are sites of carriage. Direct contact, e.g. kissing of the infected child by parents and siblings before he is removed to hospital, was undoubtedly a likely method of spread in the days when diphtheria was rife in this country and when parents were well aware that the chances of the sick child surviving were not high. Spread by fomites, e.g. drinking mugs or school pencils, has been incriminated and inhalation of dust particles contaminated with diphtheria bacilli was probably the most important mechanism of transmission.

Prevention

The remarkable reduction in incidence following on mass immunization of the community with toxoid preparations early in the Second World War underlines the high degree of protection afforded by active immunization. There is a fall-off in the proportion of people receiving such protection when the medical profession does not publicize the importance of protection to the individual and thus the community.

Isolation of cases, the administration of specific antitoxin to contacts who are not known to be protected and eradication of the carrier state all play a part in attempting to prevent the spread of diphtheria in an epidemic or potentially epidemic situation.

Corynebacterium ulcerans does not produce volutin granules but in its ability to ferment starch it resembles *gravis* strains of *C. diphtheriae*. It is, however, readily differentiated from the latter by its ability to liquefy gelatin, to produce urease and by its inability to reduce nitrates.

DIPHTHEROID BACILLI

As already stated, several members of the genus *Corynebacterium* are commensal in man.

Corynebacterium hofmannii
This occurs in the throat and like other commensal species does not produce exotoxin and is not pathogenic. More uniform in its morphology than *C. diphtheriae*, it rarely possesses volutin granules and with simple staining, e.g. with methylene blue, an unstained central bar can be seen and this is characteristic. Colonial appearances differ from those of diphtheria bacilli and Hofmann's bacillus does not ferment glucose.

Corynebacterium xerosis
This is commensal in the conjuctival sac—morphologically similar to *C. diphtheriae* but can be differentiated from the latter by its ability to ferment sucrose and in lacking pathogenicity for the guinea-pig.

Several other diphtheroid bacilli can be identified but these two are the most commonly encountered.

THE GENUS BACILLUS

Bacillus anthracis, the causative organism of anthrax, was until recently regarded as the only member of this genus pathogenic to man; however, *B. cereus* is now proven to be a cause of toxic-type food poisoning.

BACILLUS ANTHRACIS

Morphology
Large (4–8μm × 1–1·5μm), rectangular, Gram-positive bacilli with a tendency to form long strands or chains. Capsulate in the tissues and body fluids of the infected host, non-motile and forms spores when existing outside the host; characteristically the spore is oval in shape, central in position and does not project beyond the confines of the vegetative cell.

M'Fadyean's reaction
This reaction, which is characteristic of anthrax bacilli when capsulate, can be noted by microscopic examination of films of peripheral blood taken from an infected animal. The film is fixed by 1 : 1000 mercuric chloride for 5 min and then polychrome methylene blue stain is applied for 15 sec; in such a preparation the disintegrated capsules appear as

amorphous, irregular masses of heliotrope debris among which are lying large blue bacilli.

Cultural requirements
Organism grows readily on all ordinary media and over a wide temperature range (12–45°C) with an optimum for growth of 35°C. Although the vegetative cells will tolerate wide variations in their gaseous environment spore formation occurs only under aerobic conditions.

Cultural appearances
Colonies have a 'medusa-head' appearance, i.e. a wavy margin resembling locks of hair and each colony represents a continuous thread of bacilli; white, opaque and like ground-glass, some 3–4 mm in diameter after 24 hr incubation.

Biochemical activities
Anthrax bacilli ferment a variety of sugars but such tests are not employed in identifying the organism since other more striking characteristics allow easy recognition.

Serological characteristics
Several antigenic materials are now recognized and of these the exotoxin is the factor which causes death of the host. Exotoxin was discovered only a few years ago and until then it was thought that death was caused 'mechanically' by the massive septicaemic proliferation of the bacilli which block capillary blood vessels. Two somatic antigens, one a protein and the other a polysaccharide, can also be demonstrated as well as a capsular, polypeptide antigen, The latter can stimulate the formation of capsular antibody which however is without any protective effect against infection.

Animal pathogenicity
Guinea-pigs are extremely susceptible and subcutaneous injection of freshly isolated capsulate strains or of pathological material, e.g. blood from a cow dying of anthrax, results in death in 24–48 hr; the pathological picture is identical with that occurring in a naturally infected animal. There is a marked inflammatory response at the injection site with a gelatinous exudate and the local lesion is teeming with bacilli which can also be found in large numbers in the heart-blood and all organs; the spleen is particularly involved, being grossly enlarged and friable—hence the name 'splenic fever'.

Epidemiology of anthrax
Anthrax is primarily an infection of domesticated herbivorous animals but all mammals are susceptible in varying degrees; man only becomes infected by contact with sick animals or products of animals which have died from the disease.

The anthrax spore produced by vegetative cells outside the host tissues is the infecting agent in both animal and human infection. In animals, infection results usually from ingestion of the spores from contaminated pasturages where they can survive for many years. In man, anthrax is commonly a localized infection of the skin and subcutaneous tissues ('Cutaneous anthrax') and the spore gains access through a surface abrasion; certain groups of people have an occupational risk, e.g. farmers and veterinary surgeons.

Infection may result from inhalation of the spore when it contaminates wool and pulmonary anthrax in man frequently becomes septicaemic; gastrointestinal anthrax in man (clinically identical to that in animals) occurs only in the most undeveloped societies where the carcase of an anthrax-infected animal may be used as food—in such circumstances epidemics are the rule and the mortality rate is very high.

The vehicles incriminated in the spread of animal anthrax continue to expand as evidenced by the fact that in 1977 ground nuts from Senegal were shown to account for 80 outbreaks in Shropshire and neighbouring counties.

Prevention
The carcases of animals dying from anthrax must be carefully disposed of either by cremation or deep earth burial in a quick-lime pit—specific procedures are detailed in the Anthrax Orders and have the aim of limiting spore formation and the dissemination of spores. Post-mortem examination of experimentally infected laboratory animals must be made with great care to protect the operator and the total environment of the animal house. One form of cutaneous anthrax, 'Hide-porters disease', was associated with lesions across the shoulders or neck of dock porters who humped bales of contaminated hides whilst unloading ships; this was brought under control by restricting the importation of hides to one British seaport, Liverpool, and providing facilities for the mechanical handling of potentially infected material until this had undergone a rigorous disinfecting process. More recently, cutaneous anthrax has occurred sporadically and also in epidemic form in association with the use of bone-meal fertilizer containing anthrax spores and elimination of this source is under active consideration.

Pulmonary anthrax (Wool-sorter's disease) in Britain has been controlled in wool factories by carefully planned local exhaust ventilation which removes wool fibres from the air and prevents their inhalation by workers.

Gastrointestinal anthrax in humans can be readily prevented by ensuring that man cannot have access to anthrax carcases. Various kinds of vaccine are available for active immunization of animals; spore vaccines prepared from non-capsulate virulent strains have been used successfully in many countries but are not used to protect humans since they are considered not to be sufficiently safe. Individuals following occupations with a high risk of infection can be actively immunized with a vaccine made from the somatic protein antigen; its protective value against cutaneous anthrax is satisfactory.

OTHER MEMBERS OF THE GENUS BACILLUS

Bacillus cereus has the usual features of the genus but is readily differentiated from *B. anthracis* by producing haemolysis on blood agar and by the fact that it is not lysed by specific (gamma) phage.

The popular association of cases and epidemics of toxic-type food poisoning caused by *B. cereus* with fried rice is justified on present epidemiological evidence; however, the ubiquitous nature of *B. cereus* is emphasized when we note that other plant foods are incriminated in the syndrome.

The usual epidemiological picture is that rice grains are parboiled and instead of being fried within 1–4 hr they are left at room temperature, e.g. overnight; thus spores of *B. cereus* which survive parboiling can germinate and the vegetative cells grow on the partly cooked rice and elaborate one or both of enterotoxins A and B which can tolerate the brief exposure to frying temperatures and cause either an essentially diarrhoeal or vomiting type syndrome

This again serves to emphasize the golden rule *that foodstuffs should be eaten immediately after being prepared and cooked, or alternatively, they should be immediately stored at temperatures which prevent bacterial multiplication.*

There are numerous saprophytic species in this genus and these are collectively referred to as anthracoid bacilli. They are ubiquitous and are frequently encountered as contaminants in the laboratory. Their occurrence need not create any difficulties in differentiation from anthrax bacilli since, unlike the latter, they do not give a M'Fadyean reaction and are non-pathogenic for guinea-pigs when administered in doses similar to those of *B. anthracis*. Many of the saprophytic species are motile and give marked haemolysis on blood agar in comparison with the feeble haemolytic activity of the anthrax bacillus.

CHAPTER 17
Anaerobic Gram-positive bacilli

LACTOBACILLI

Morphology
Classically the cells are large, 1–5μm × 1μm, and appear as pairs or short chains but pleomorphism predominates in old cultures. Non-sporing, non-motile and non-capsulate.

Cultural requirements
Grow over a wide temperature range, 15–45°C, although some species are more restricted; optimum = 37°C. Prefer aciduric conditions, i.e. at about pH 5·8. Prefer anaerobic conditions and some species are strict anaerobes. Growth is slow but is enhanced by the addition to nutrient agar of glucose or yeast extract.

Cultural appearances
After incubation at 37°C under anaerobic conditions for 2–4 days colonies are 0·5 mm in diameter usually with an irregular edge and a granular appearance.

Biochemical activities
Fifteen species can be identified from their varying actions on a wide range of carbohydrate substrates but only a few have significance in human medicine.

Serological characteristics
Although serotypes can be identified within species using agglutinating antisera such procedures are not undertaken routinely in diagnostic laboratories.

103

Occurrence
Lactobacilli occur widely in nature, leading a saprophytic existence
and are also commonly commensal on man and animals. Within a day
or two of birth the alimentary canal is colonized from the mother and
in health lactobacilli are among the most numerous commensal
bacterial species; the commonest species is *Lactobacillus acidophilus*
and colonization of the gut is lifelong although the bowel population
of lactobacilli can be quite dramatically reduced when certain broad
spectrum antibiotics are given to the patient.

Another site where lactobacilli present as the predominating commensal species is the vagina during the productive years of a woman's
life; here the lactobacilli utilize the glycogen of the vaginal cells and the
production of lactic acid results in the vaginal secretions having a pH
of approximately 4·5; such a milieu explains in large part the virtual
freedom from infection of the vagina during the childbearing years.

Dental caries
Lactobacilli undoubtedly participate in the production of dental caries
which is of multifactorial origin; their role appears to be the continued
invasion and destruction of the tooth after the primary attack on the
enamel and dentine in which salivary streptococci play a major part.

CLOSTRIDIA

Anaerobic spore-bearing Gram-positive bacilli are collectively members
of the genus *Clostridium*. There are numerous species and the majority
lead a saprophytic existence and play an important role in the decom-
position of dead animal and plant life; some occur commensally in the
intestinal tract of man and animals and a few produce potentially lethal
diseases in man—-botulism, tetanus and gas gangrene.

CL. BOTULINUM

Morphology
Straight-sided rods with rounded ends, measuring approximately
$4\mu m \times 1\mu m$. Non-capsulate, motile with a peritrichous flagellar dis-
tribution, spores are oval, subterminal and projecting.

Cultural requirements
Strict anaerobe, temperature range for growth is 20–37°C, optimum is
35°C; grows on ordinary media.

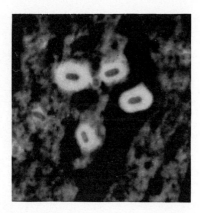

PLATE 1. Wet Indian ink film of a strain of *Klebsiella aerogenes* showing capsules and loose slime. × 1600.

Four bacilli can be seen and each is surrounded by a large capsule; the capsulate bacilli are on a background of loose slime which is partly infiltrated by carbon particles of the ink so that the slime is slightly darker than the bacterial capsules.

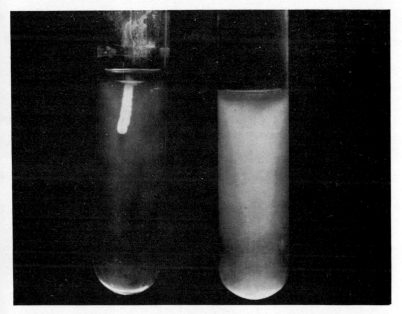

PLATE 2. Motility testing in semi-solid agar. The tube of semi-solid agar on the left was inoculated by means of a straight wire to a depth of ½ in. with a non-motile organism; the tube of semi-solid agar on the right was similarly inoculated but with a motile organism. After incubation at 37°C for 18 hours it can be noted that the growth of the non-motile organism was restricted to the original inoculum track; in contrast, the motile organisms have spread throughout the medium and the inoculum track is not visible.

PLATE 3 From Passmore & Robson (1970) *A Companion to Medical Studies,* Vol. 2. Oxford: Blackwell Scientific Publications.

(a) These two photographs are of the same pure culture of *Corynebacterium diphtheriae*; the upper preparation has been stained by Gram's method and the lower by Albert's staining method to demonstrate the presence of volutin granules (× 1000).

(b) Tellurite blood agar medium which had been inoculated with *C. diphtheriae* var. *intermedius* 36 hours previously and incubated at 37°C. This medium is very selective for diphtheria bacilli and allied species; on it the three biotypes of *C. diphtheriae* give rise to different colonies that an experienced bacteriologist can distinguish.

(e) This Gram-stained preparation is from a culture of *Actinomyces israelii*, the causal organism of human actinomycosis; the long branching filaments, showing some fragmentation, emerge from a dense mycelium (× 1000).

(f) Film from a pure culture of *Clostridium tetani* and stained by Ziehl–Neelsen's method modified by using a weaker strength of H_2SO_4 (0·5 per cent) for decolourization; the terminal, spherical and projecting spores produce the typical appearance of 'the drumstick bacillus' (× 1000).

(i) Film stained for 10 min with 1 in 10 carbol fuchsin; the film was from a case of gingivostomatitis and shows large numbers of *Fusiformis fusiformis* (cigar-shaped bacilli) and *Borrelia vincentii* (spirochaetes) (× 1000).

(j) Carbol fuchsin-stained film of blood from a white mouse that had been infected with *Borrelia duttonii*, the cause of West African relapsing fever (× 1000).

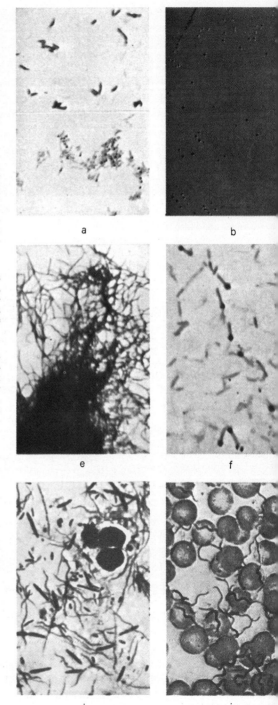

a

b

e

f

i

j

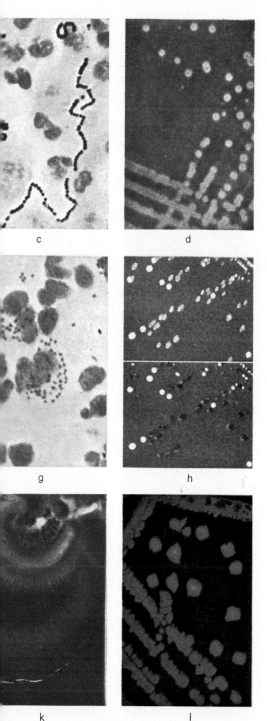

c

d

g

h

k

l

(c) Film of pus containing *Streptococcus pyogenes*. Chains of varying length are apparent, but the chain length is no guide to the cultural type of streptococcus. Gram stain (× 1000).

(d) Blood agar plate seeded with a throat swab and incubated for 18 hours at 37°C. Two colonial types of streptococci are present; these are identical in size but β-haemolysis around the colonies of the pathogenic *Strept. pyogenes* makes them more obvious than the colonies of commensal *Strept. viridans* which form a series of α-haemolytic spots in the background.

(g) Film of urethral discharge from a case of gonorrhoea; two polymorphs are packed with Gram-positive diplococci. This intracellular appearance is characteristic of the pathogenic neisseriae (× 1000).

(h) Chocolate blood agar medium seeded with urethral discharge and incubated for 48 hours at 37°C in air with 5 per cent CO_2. The white, pigmented colonies were shown to be coagulase-negative staphylococci; the lower photograph was taken 5 sec after oxidase reagent had been flooded over the plate. The colonies that then became purple belong to the genus *Neisseria* and biochemical tests showed that they were *N. gonorrhoeae*.

(k) This blood agar plate was stab-inoculated with a pure culture of *Proteus vulgaris* and then incubated at 37°C for 18 hours; successive waves of spreading growth can be seen. The swarming nature of *Proteus* species frequently delays the isolation of other species in mixed culture but can be prevented by incorporating various substances, e.g. chloral hydrate (1 in 500), in the medium.

(l) This nutrient agar plate was seeded with a swab from an infected burn and then incubated at 37°C for 18 hours; the natural light straw colour of the medium has been altered by pyocyanin pigment produced by the organism.

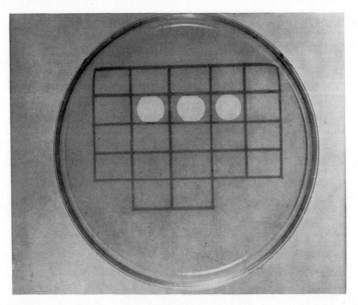

PLATE 4. Phage-typing of staphyiococci. A grid of 22 oblongs was marked on the outer surface of this Petri dish which contained digest agar and each oblong corresponds to the site of one phage preparation. The surface of the agar was flooded with a broth culture of coagulase-positive staphylococci and after the plate had dried 22 phage preparations were applied individually; after these preparations had dried, the plate was incubated at 37°C for 18 hours. Examination of the plate revealed confluent lysis of the staphylococcal lawn at three sites corresponding to the areas of phage preparations 3B, 3C and 55.

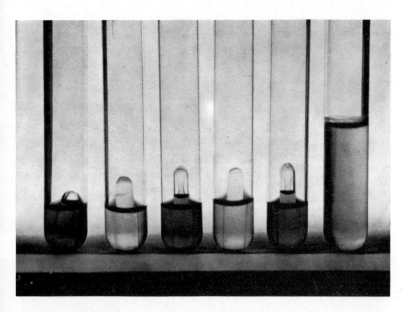

PLATE 5. The inoculum for this set of sugars and the tube of peptone water was a pale, lactose non-fermenting colony from a DCA plate. The sugars are respectively from left to right, glucose, lactose, dulcite, sucrose and mannite. Glucose, dulcite and mannite have been fermented and with gas production as noted in the small Durham tubes. Indole was not produced in the peptone water culture but the organisms were motile; on this evidence the culture was potentially a member of the genus *Salmonella* and subsequent serological investigation proved the isolate to be *S. paratyphi B*.

PLATE 6 From Passmore & Robson (1970) *A Companion to Medical Studies*, vol. 2. Oxford: Blackwell Scientific Publications.

(a) Film of pus containing staphylococci showing the characteristic arrangement. Gram stain (× 1000).

(b) Blood agar plate seeded with pus and incubated at 37°C for 18 hours; a pure and profuse growth of *Staphylococcus aureus* is seen. These proved to be coagulase-positive (plate 6k); the colonies should be contrasted with the smaller, non-pigmented colonies of streptococci in plate 3d.

(e) Film of sputum from a case of lobar pneumonia. The pneumococci occur in pairs; the capsules are not demonstrated by the Gram stain (× 1000).

(f) Blood agar plate seeded with a pure culture of pneumococci and incubated for 36 hours at 37°C; the colonial size after 18 hours was identical with that of *Strept. viridans* in plate 3d and the associated α-haemolysis was similar.

(i) Gram-stained film of a pure culture of *Escherichia coli*; these are indistinguishable from other enterobacteria by Gram staining.

(j) The culture medium employed here is that of MacConkey which contains lactose and phenol red indicator; in the upper half is a mixed culture of *Esch. coli* showing pink, lactose-fermenting colonies with pale, lactose non-fermenting colonies which proved to be *Shigella sonnei*. In the lower part are colonies of *Klebsiella aerogenes* which have also utilized the lactose; this species produces large amounts of extracellular slime which endows the colonies with a mucoid appearance and also allows adjacent colonies to coalesce.

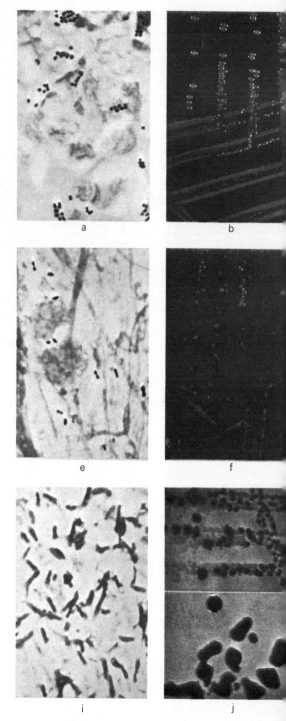

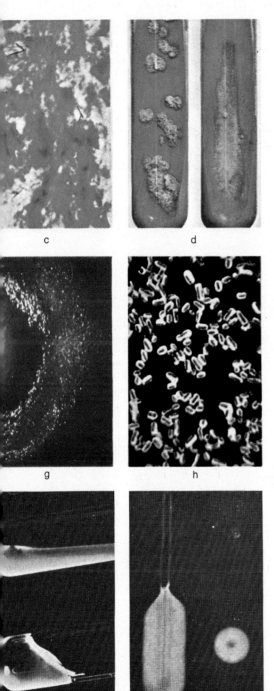

c

d

g

h

k

l

(c) Film of a concentrated specimen of sputum stained by the Ziehl–Neelsen method; acid- and alcohol-fast bacilli can be noted against the background debris which has been counter-stained with methylene blue (× 1000).

(d) Lowenstein–Jensen egg medium. On the left is the appearance of human type tubercle bacilli, *Mycobacterium tuberculosis*, after 8 weeks' incubation at 37°C; such growth is often described as being 'rough, tough and buff' in comparison with the smooth, friable and whitish appearance of bovine type bacilli, *Myco. bovis*, as shown on the right. The latter culture had been incubated under identical conditions and illustrates the slow growth of these mycobacteria even on rich media.

(g) Blood agar plate viewed by oblique illumination in an endeavour to show the very fine, diaphanous film of spreading growth characteristic of *Cl. tetani*.

(h) Preparation of *Clostridium welchii* showing capsules; this India ink film was dried, fixed with methanol and then stained with methyl violet for 2 min. For normal purposes, India ink films are viewed in the wet state.

(k) Coagulase tests. Both tubes contained citrated rabbit plasma, diluted 1 in 10 in sterile saline; the upper tube received five drops of an overnight broth culture of a non-pathogenic staphylococcus and the lower tube received a similar volume of a broth culture of a staphylococcus isolated from an infected wound. The tubes were then incubated overnight at 37°C for 6 hours. The contents of the upper tube remained fluid, whereas the plasma in the lower tube has been gelled; thus the staphylococcus inoculated into the latter tube was coagulase-positive.

(l) Nagler's reaction on egg-yolk medium. Three drops of *Clostridium welchii* type-A antiserum were spread over one-half (upper part of plate) of the medium; a culture of *Cl. welchii* was then streaked on the medium and two spot inoculations were also made. After anaerobic incubation at 37°C for 20 hours, the organisms grew on both halves of the plate. On the antitoxin-free half, lecithinase activity produced zones of opacity but this activity has been inhibited by the antitoxin present on the upper half.

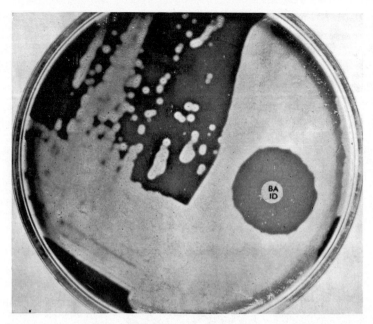

PLATE 7. This crystal violet blood agar plate was inoculated from a throat swab. A bacitracin disk was placed in the well inoculum area and after incubation for 18 hours at 37°C a pure growth of β-haemolytic streptococci was noted; the growth was sensitive to bacitracin which indicates that the strain belonged to Lancefield's group A (*Strept. pyogenes*). Occasionally bacitracin-sensitive strains belong to group C or G.

Cultural appearances
Considerable variation but colonies often have an irregular edge and those of toxin-producing strains are semi-transparent whereas the colonies of non-toxigenic sporing variants are opaque.

Biochemical activities
The six antigenically distinct types show variation in their saccharolytic and proteolytic activities, but details of these are not necessary for our present purposes.

Serological characteristics
The six types (A–F) produce antigenically distinct exotoxins and each of these neurotoxins can be neutralized only by its own antitoxin and this allows us to establish the type of any strain isolated.

Animal pathogenicity
Guinea-pigs and other laboratory animals when challenged by inoculation or by feeding with cultures are susceptible and clinically suffer an illness similar to that in man; animals may be protected with specific antitoxins so that we can demonstrate the type of neurotoxin produced by an isolate.

Epidemiology of botulism
Although every type has been incriminated, in human cases types A, B and E are most frequently involved. The organisms are saprophytic and can be isolated from soil, fruit, vegetables, etc.; man is affected by ingesting foodstuffs in which the organisms have had time to form their exotoxin and almost all reported outbreaks have been associated with *preserved* foods of various kinds. Botulism is essentially an *intoxication* and not an infection—secondary cases are rare, if they occur at all.

Prevention
The food *industry* is well aware of the danger of botulism and precautions are taken to ensure that foodstuffs are heated sufficiently to destroy even the spores of *Cl. botulinum*; *home* preservation of foods is much more risky as is reflected by the seasonal incidence in North America where most cases occur during the winter months when such home-preserved foods are consumed more frequently and in larger quantities than at any other season.

Antitoxin may be administered to individuals who may have eaten food which is suspect; active immunization is possible with a mixed

toxoid preparation but is not justified in countries where the disease is
rare.

CL. TETANI

Morphology
Straight, rod-shaped and measuring approximately $5\mu m \times 0\cdot5\mu m$; motile
with peritrichous flagella, non-capsulate. Spores are spherical, terminal
and projecting and for this reason the organism is referred to as the
'drum-stick bacillus' but it is not unique in this regard.

   Cl. tetanomorphum displays spores identical in size, shape and
position to those of *Cl. tetani* but the former species is non-pathogenic.

Cultural requirements
Strict anaerobe and even established *in vitro* cultures die rapidly on
exposure to the normal atmosphere; wide temperature range for growth
14–42°C, optimum 37°C. Grows on ordinary media but growth is enhanced if blood is incorporated.

Cultural appearances
Discrete colonies are not usually seen and growth is characterized by a
fine diaphanous film from the edges of which extend numerous long
branching projections. Non-motile variants give rise to isolated colonies
which rarely exceed 1 mm in diameter and are transparent with an
entire circular edge devoid of any projection.

Biochemical activities
No saccharolytic activity; slight proteolytic action as shown by minimal
digestion of meat particles in cooked-meat broth.

Serological characteristics
Ten types of *Cl. tetani* can be distinguished on the basis of flagellar
antigens but all ten serotypes produce an identical exotoxin; certain
strains in each serotype may be non-toxigenic.

Animal pathogenicity
In addition to man, several animals are naturally susceptible to tetanus
and in the laboratory mice are employed for diagnostic purposes. As in
similar animal tests with other bacteria or their toxins, a pair of animals
is used in each test and one of the pair is protected with tetanus antitoxin before both are challenged. Unprotected mice inoculated intramuscularly in a hind leg show evidence of tetanus within a few hours;
the tail stiffens and the inoculated limb becomes paralysed. Paralysis

then becomes generalized and tetanic spasms occur on the slightest stimulus.

Epidemiology of tetanus
In contrast to *Cl. botulinum* which can be isolated from virgin soil and therefore leads a truly saprophytic existence, it is not certain that tetanus bacilli are also saprophytic; the soil population may be derived from faecal contamination by animals and man and certainly the organisms are most prevalent in soil which has been manured.

Almost invariably tetanus spores enter a wound by means of soil contamination; occasionally catgut, made from sheep's intestines, is inadequately processed and has acted as a source of infection in surgical wounds. The mere presence of spores in a wound does not invariably result in clinical tetanus since their germination is dependent on various factors; devitalized tissue, the presence of foreign material such as soil or clothing and the coexistence of aerobic organisms are factors which contribute to a reduction in oxygen tension around spores and allow them to germinate as well as encouraging the growth of the vegetative cells which emerge. Toxin-producing strains present in a wound remain restricted to the site of wounding and the clinical picture is caused by the effects of the neurotoxin which diffuses to the nervous system.

Tetanus does not spread directly from man to man and when epidemics occur they are due to several individuals being infected from a common source.

Prevention
Emergency prophylaxis in the non-immunized individual depends on early and thorough surgical treatment of the wound combined with the administration of tetanus antitoxin. Alternatively, penicillin can be given prophylactically if the patient has a history of hypersensitivity to horse serum.

The comparatively recent introduction of human tetanus immuno-globulin for passive immunization has eliminated the hazard associated with the older horse serum antitoxin. Thus, human tetanus immuno-globulin should be given to injured people who have not been actively immunized with toxoid and simultaneously, but at a different ana-tomical site, tetanus toxoid should be administered to start the active immunization programme.

Long-term protection, particularly to groups at special risk, e.g. farm workers, depends on active immunization with tetanus toxoid; the basic course of immunization comprises three injections each of 0·5 ml of toxoid with a 6-weeks interval between the first two, the third injection being given some 6–12 months after the second dose.

The reduction in incidence of tetanus neonatorum in more primitive societies is essentially dependent on education in safe methods of dressing the umbilical stump, since there is little doubt that a dressing of cow-dung is the usual vehicle for tetanus spores.

Obviously, cat-gut, dressings, umbilical-cord powder and other materials used in wound dressing and surgical procedures must be free from tetanus spores.

CL. WELCHII

This species is by far the most commonly incriminated in cases of gas-gangrene in man, either as sole agent or in combination with other members of the genus, e.g. *Cl. oedematiens* and *Cl. septicum*.

Morphology
Bacilli have rounded or square ends and measure approximately $5\mu m \times 1\mu m$. Unlike all other clostridia, *Cl. welchii* is *non-motile*. Forms capsules in animal tissues but not on *in vitro* cultivation. Spores are sub-terminal, oval and non-projecting.

Cultural requirements
Anaerobic but not as strictly so as *Cl. tetani*; grows rapidly at 37°C but particularly if a fermentable carbohydrate, e.g. glucose, is incorporated in the culture medium.

Cultural appearances
While there is some variation in colonial morphology, colonies are usually large (3–5 mm), semi-opaque with an entire edge, and on blood agar β-haemolysis is usually evident.

Biochemical activities
Ferments a variety of sugars, e.g. glucose, lactose and maltose, with production of gas. In litmus milk medium *Cl. welchii* produces acid with clotting of the medium and gas, produced from fermentation of the lactose, disrupts the clot resulting in the 'stormy clot reaction'.

Serological characteristics
Five types (A–E) of *Cl. welchii* can be identified according to the types of major lethal toxins they produce; type A strains are most commonly pathogenic for man and these produce only the alpha toxin, whereas

types B–E, which are usually associated with disease in various animals produce in addition one or more of the beta, epsilon and iota toxins.

Nagler's Reaction. Alpha toxin is an enzyme, lecithinase C, and its antitoxin is highly specific. When a strain producing lecithinase is grown on an egg yolk medium a zone of opalescence surrounds the growth and this precipitation can be inhibited if alpha antitoxin is present. This is known as Nagler's reaction and is performed by spreading the antitoxin over one half of the surface of the medium, before streak inoculation of the organism is made, so that it will grow on both halves of the medium. It is important to inoculate the plate from the untreated half to the antitoxin half, otherwise antitoxin might be carried over to the normal surface.

Animal pathogenicity
Strains vary greatly in their pathogenicity; pathogenic strains injected intramuscularly kill guinea-pigs within 24–48 hr. An hour or two after injection oedema occurs in the injected leg and gas formation allows elicitation of crepitation in the tissues; oedema and tissue destruction spread rapidly and the organisms can be recovered from the heart-blood 8–12 hr after injection. Animals injected with specific antitoxin prior to challenge with a culture show no ill effects.

Epidemiology of gas-gangrene
Cl. welchii is a normal inhabitant of the large intestine of animals and man, thus manured soil or other materials in which spores may exist, e.g. clothing, act as a plentiful reservoir. Thus, as in the case of tetanus, a wound may be contaminated and gas-gangrene might result. Detailed study of wounds during the Second World War revealed that many wounds in which pathogenic species were present healed without any evidence of gas-gangrene and in others, although the disease was present in the injured muscle, it did not invade healthy muscle in the same limb and this localized infection is referred to as anaerobic cellulitis. Finally, classical gas-gangrene may occur when organisms display their full invasive ability and spread very rapidly into healthy muscle which then undergoes toxic necrosis.

Of the several other members of the genus which are incriminated in gas-gangrene, *Cl. oedematiens*, *Cl. septicum* and *Cl. bifermentans* occur most commonly; these strains can be differentiated from each other and from *Cl. welchii* biochemically and by serological methods.

Prevention

Prophylaxis is primarily dependent on *thorough surgical treatment* of a wound soon after injury. Ancillary preventive measures include the administration of suitable antibiotics and although the infection is rare in civilian life, the administration of antitoxic serum should not be withheld in severe wounds which might be liable to gas-gangrene. Polyvalent serum is given if the organisms have not been isolated and monovalent serum when specific identification has been made.

One particular situation where per-operative penicillin prophylaxis is mandatory is in the amputation of the lower limb at any level, and especially where the blood supply to the limb is jeopardized.

CHAPTER 18
Gram-negative bacilli, I

The family *Enterobacteriaceae* contains many genera and apart from the fact that some are motile and others are not *they are morphologically* indistinguishable.

Morphology of enterobacteria
Size variable, but approximately 3–5μm × 0·5μm, relatively straight cells with rounded ends, some species may be capsulate and some possess fimbriae. None produces spores.

ESCHERICHIA COLI
The majority of strains are motile.

Cultural requirements
Grows over a wide temperature range—15–41°C, optimum 37°C; also tolerant of atmospheric conditions. Grows well on ordinary media.

Cultural appearances
On nutrient agar, colonies are large, 2–4 mm in diameter after 18 hr at 37°C; opacity of colonies varies with different strains but all are convex and with an entire edge. On MacConkey's medium colonies are similar to those on agar but are rose-pink since lactose is fermented; *Esch. coli* do not grow well on deoxycholate-citrate-agar (DCA) and colonies are small and pink.

Biochemical activities
Like most other enterobacteria, *Esch. coli* has a wide range of activity on many substrates. However, the bacteriologist engaged in diagnostic

111

work makes use of only a few tests which allow him to differentiate *Esch. coli* strains from microscopically similar species which, in the same site, may be pathogenic, e.g. *Esch. coli* almost invariably ferment lactose whereas salmonella and shigella strains cannot do so; similarly indole production by *Esch. coli* differentiates them from salmonella species.

Serological characteristics

Strains can be serotyped for epidemiological purposes by identification of somatic and flagellar antigens with relevant specific antisera. However, most interest centres around the K (Kapsule) antigens, which are present in certain strains which can cause gastroenteritis. These K antigens of which three types, L, A and B, can be differentiated, reside on the surface of strains either in a recognizable capsule or as an envelope which is too fine to be seen.

Epidemiology of *Esch. coli* infection

Esch. coli is essentially a commensal of the intestinal tract of animals and man and thus it is widely distributed in the environment.

Endogenous infection of the urinary tract is the usual type of infection caused by such strains but they are also involved in peritonitis, appendix abscess and wound infections either alone, or with other organisms, e.g. enterococci.

Exogenous infection of the urinary tract also occurs and the organisms are usually introduced during catheterization either on inadequately sterilized instruments or because of a breakdown in aseptic technique.

Gastroenteritis resulting from infection with enteropathogenic strains of *Esch. coli* is not restricted to any age group but is most commonly seen in epidemic form in infants; the source of such strains may be a carrier or a case of infection and the higher incidence among artificially-fed babies emphasizes that spread from the source is often by means of contaminated milk-feeds.

Prevention

In exogenously acquired infection of the urinary tract, wounds, etc. prophylaxis depends on adequate sterilization of instruments, dressings, and other materials and thorough aseptic procedures in operating and dressings rooms and in the ward.

Terminal heat-treatment of feeds for infants can eliminate the major method of spread of gastroenteritis but, in addition, the mother and hospital personnel must be rigorous in their personal hygiene. In the domestic situation the mother should be advised to prepare a feed immediately before use and should be instructed in the aseptic handling of the feeding bottle and the raw materials in preparing the feed.

PROTEUS

The morphology and cultural requirements of members of this genus are very similar to those of *Esch. coli*. Almost all strains are motile.

Cultural appearances
On nutrient agar, isolated colonies are only occasionally seen and these are similar to those of *Esch. coli*; usually *Proteus* species swarm over the surface of the medium in successive waves. Since non-motile variants do not swarm the phenomenon is obviously associated with motility but its exact cause is not known.

Swarming can be inhibited if the strain is grown on MacConkey's medium or if one of several agents, e.g. 1 in 500 chloral hydrate, is added to the medium. Swarming has a nuisance value to the bacteriologist since the sheet of growth may cover colonies of other significant organisms.

Biochemical activities
Four biochemical types of *Proteus* can be recognized and all are readily differentiated from other enterobacteria by their ability to produce urease; although some other members of the family *Enterobacteriaceae* can decompose urea, none can do so as quickly as the *Proteus* species.

Serological characteristics
All four biochemical types can be further subdivided by agglutination reactions into many groups and serotypes depending respectively on their somatic and flagellar antigens but serotyping is not performed routinely.

The specific nature of the reaction between an antigen and its antibody has been referred to in Chapter 6 but one of the few exceptions in specificity of such reactions concerns certain types of *Proteus* which have antigens identical with some rickettsiae. These types are used as antigens in agglutination tests with serum from patients suspected of suffering from rickettsial infection, e.g. the Weil-Felix reaction in cases of typhus fever.

Epidemiology and prevention of Proteus infections
With the exception that *Proteus* species do not cause gastroenteritis, the
sources and methods of spread of infection caused by them are identical
to those of *Esch. coli.*

SHIGELLAE

All members of the genus *Shigella* are non-motile but otherwise are
identical in morphology and cultural requirements with *Esch. coli.*

Cultural appearances
These resemble those of *Esch. coli* except that they do not ferment
lactose and the colonies are therefore pale or colourless; members of
one group, i.e. *Sh. sonnei*, are late lactose fermenters thus, after incubation on MacConkey's or DCA medium for 24 hr or more, their colonies
have a light pink appearance.

Biochemical activities
Four biochemical groups of shigella can be recognized:

	Glucose	Lactose	Mannitol	Indole
Sh. dysenteriae	⊥	—	—	V
Sh. flexneri	⊥	—	⊥	V
Sh. boydii	⊥	—	⊥	V
Sh. sonnei	⊥	(⊥)	⊥	⊥

⊥ = acid produced; no gas.   (⊥) = late reaction.
V = variable reaction   — = no reaction.

   With the exception of certain strains of *Sh. flexneri* serotype 6, no
gas is produced in fermentation reactions.

Serological characteristics
Each biochemical group is antigenically distinctive and with the exception of *Sh. sonnei* each can be subdivided into several serotypes and in
the case of certain *Sh. flexneri* strains subtypes can also be recognized.

Epidemiology of bacillary dysentery
Members of the genus *Shigella* are parasites of man and of a few
higher apes. Infection is by ingestion, and to some extent the severity

of clinical illness is associated with the particular group to which the organism belongs, tending to be more serious when *Sh. dysenteriae* strains are involved whilst in the case of *Sh. sonnei* infection, a mild, short illness is the rule.

In countries or areas with inadequate sewage disposal systems, flies and other insects may feed on human excreta and then soil foodstuffs, but in more sophisticated countries insects do not play a role and methods of spread from a human case or carrier is 'hand-to-mouth'. Direct contact as in hand-shaking and indirect contact via toilet fixtures and door handles is the usual method of transmission.

In Britain, where for many years Sonne dysentery has predominated and increased in incidence, the disease can be used as an index of personal hygiene; the mild nature of Sonne dysentery allows many cases to remain ambulant and thus to act as peripatetic disseminators.

Prevention

In Britain it is probable that improved personal hygiene, particularly hand-washing after defaecation and before handling food, could greatly reduce the spread of Sonne dysentery. Even then, the use of communal towels would allow the transmission of the organisms from person to person so individual towels made of paper or other materials should replace roller-towels. Of course, in areas where flies have access to faeces physical and chemical fly-control methods should be employed to protect foodstuffs.

Perhaps one of the factors contributing to the increasing incidence of Sonne dysentery in the past was the fact that, until recently, no method of typing the serologically homogeneous *Sh. sonnei* was available. Colicine typing allows the recognition of at least 17 epidemiologically significant types and this typing method should encourage more detailed investigation of outbreaks. No vaccines are available for active immunization.

Colicine typing depends on the detection of various patterns of bacteriocine production on a standard set of indicator strains.

The strain to be typed is seeded as a heavily inoculated diametric streak on the surface of a tryptone soya blood agar plate which is then incubated at 35°C for 24 hr. This incubation temperature is vital if reliable and replicable results are to be obtained. Thereafter the macroscopic growth of the producer strain is scraped off the surface and microscopic elements are sterilized by exposure to chloroform vapour for a few minutes.

The indicator strains, 15 in number, are then inoculated on to the medium at right angles to the line of the original inoculum and the plates are incubated at 37°C for 18 hr.

Bacteriocines produced by the primary inoculum will variously inhibit different indicator strains and allow the recognition of colicine types from the various patterns of inhibition. A similar technique is used in pyocine typing of *Pseudomonas pyocyanea*.

SALMONELLAE

With two exceptions all of the 1800 or more serotypes of salmonellae are motile; their morphology and cultural requirements are very similar to those of *Esch. coli*.

Cultural appearances
Salmonellae resembles closely the pale colourless colonies of shigellae.

Biochemical activities
Salmonellae are variously active on many substrates and with the exception of *S. typhi* fermentation is accompanied by gas production. For preliminary identification it is usual to show that glucose, dulcitol and mannitol are fermented and that a strain does not utilize lactose or sucrose and that indole is not produced.

Subsequent confirmation of identity is by serological methods but some serotypes, e.g. *S. enteritidis*, can be subdivided into epidemiologically significant varieties by extended tests of their biochemical ability.

Serological characteristics
A salmonella isolated from pathological material can be allocated to one of several *groups* by identifying its *somatic* antigens with group-specific antisera; the *type* identification within any one group depends on the use of highly type-specific *flagellar* antisera. There are potential complicating factors in both grouping and typing procedures. Firstly, a few salmonellae, e.g. *S. typhi*, have a third antigen, namely the Vi (virulence) antigen which occurs as a surface coating and masks agglutination with somatic antisera; before the somatic antigen can be recognized a suspension of the Vi-possessing strain must be boiled for 1 hr and then washed by centrifuging.

Secondly, the flagellar antigens of any one species may be present in either or both of two phases; phase 1 antigen is specific for its own type species, whereas phase 2 antigen is non-specific and is shared with many species; thus an isolate must be in the specific phase 1 state before it can be typed.

Isolates which are found to be in the non-specific phase, i.e. the *majority* of the culture population possesses phase 2 antigen, can usually be obtained in the specific phase by using Craigie's tube method, which employs semi-solid agar to which has been added phase 2 anti-serum (1 in 50). Within the main container is placed an open-ended piece of glass tubing which projects above the surface of the medium; when phase 2 organisms are inoculated in the agar *within* the glass tubing and incubated they are agglutinated by the phase 2 antiserum and immobilized. Only phase 1 organisms, which are in the minority in the inoculum, remain motile and can thus spread from the inner tube and escape from its lower end into the medium outside the tube. Thus by taking sub-cultures from the surface of the medium *outside* the inner tube one can harvest specific phase bacilli.

Epidemiology of Salmonella infections
Salmonellae can cause either the enteric fevers, i.e. typhoid and para-typhoid fever, or food poisoning and these differ in many respects.

Enteric fevers
These are caused by *S. typhi* and the three types *A*, *B* and *C* of *S. para-typhi*. Human cases and carriers are the only sources of infection and in the case of typhoid fever the spread from a human source is classically by means of water supplies; however, foodstuffs also act as vehicles of infection in the enteric fevers. *S. paratyphi B* is the type most commonly encountered in Britain.

After ingestion the organisms reach the small intestine and pass by lymphatic spread to the mesenteric glands where they multiply and then, via the thoracic duct, invade the blood stream. Only at this stage does the patient become a source of infection and increasingly so as the bacteraemic phase comes to an end. During the bacteraemic phase many tissues are invaded including the liver, gall bladder and kidneys; from the gall bladder a second invasion of the intestine takes place and on this occasion obvious pathological effects occur with particular involvement of the lymphoid tissue, the bacilli being excreted in large numbers in the faeces. Similarly, if the organisms become localized in the kidney they will be excreted in the urine.

In approximately 3% of patients excretion continues after clinical recovery and although carriage is often temporary it may continue indefinitely. In chronic carriage the bacilli are usually present in the gall bladder or less commonly in the urinary tract. Cases of enteric fever which are recognized and treated in isolation are not as great a danger to the community as are carriers. Apart from the risk of contaminating water supplies, carriers may contaminate foodstuffs with bacilli which are present on their hands and many foodstuffs have thus been incriminated as vehicles of infection.

As in bacillary dysentery, insects may act as vectors of spread if they have access to infected faeces.

Salmonella food poisoning
In comparison with the enteric fevers the incubation period of salmonella food poisoning is short (1–2 days as against 10–14 days), the clinical illness is brief and lasts only a week or less, infection is often localized to the gut, and bacteraemia is not a constant finding and man is not the only source of infection. Domestic animals, e.g. cattle, sheep and pigs, and also fowls can suffer infection and also act as carriers; similarly rodents are a constant potential source of infection.

A carrier rate of 1% has been found in healthy beef cattle and sheep and it has been shown that this rate increases as animals are moved from farms to abattoirs, especially if the transit period is lengthy and/or the animals are overcrowded in trucks and are not given a plentiful supply of food and water.

Carcases can obviously become contaminated at any stage during marketing or during preparation for human consumption in butchers' premises, hotel and other kitchens either from other carcases, from human cases or carriers or from the excreta of rats and mice.

Intensive farming techniques undoubtedly increase the risk of animals transmitting infection to each other and hence increase the danger to the human population. This situation is even more unhappy if the animals are fed with foodstuffs containing antibiotics in an endeavour to increase their beef yield and hence their market value. Thus salmonella strains in such animals can and do develop resistance to antibiotics which otherwise might be useful in treating the person ultimately suffering infection.

Milk and milk products may also be a source of infection, as can hen and duck eggs; if these are pooled or used in making custards etc., which will be communally consumed then several individuals will be at risk. On the other hand, many cases of individual infection are probably undetected when an egg is eaten by one person.

Prevention of enteric fevers

Measures which are generally enforceable include the provision and maintenance of safe water supplies and adequate water-borne sewage systems, supervision of workers in water-works and in the food industry, protection of foodstuffs from insects and bacteriological control of imported foodstuffs. Similarly the prompt isolation and treatment of all cases is required and known carriers must not be employed in any situation where they might contaminate water or food.

Specifically, people at special risk, e.g. troops or travellers in areas where the disease is endemic, can be offered a reasonable degree of protection by active immunization with phenolized TAB vaccine; for people living in Britain, only those living with chronic carriers and laboratory personnel working with specimens or live suspensions need be offered immunization.

Prevention of Salmonella food poisoning

Human cases and carriers must obviously be prevented from working in any situation where they might contaminate articles of food and drink, including such articles intended for animal consumption; infected animals must speedily be withdrawn from the herd or flock and killed.

Abattoirs, wholesale and retail butchers' shops and other premises where food is prepared or cooked should be maintained in a clean state and such premises should be rodent-proof and fly-proof.

Wherever possible food should be eaten immediately after cooking but when this is impracticable it must be stored in refrigerators so that any organisms which have survived can at least be prevented from multiplying. The education of food-handlers in the need for a high level of personal hygiene and in methods of handling foodstuffs so that contamination is minimal is a very important aspect of prophylaxis. No protective vaccines are available.

KLEBSIELLAE

Morphology

Size, shape and response to Gram's staining method are identical to other enterobacteria; non-motile, non-sporing but usually are capsulate *in vivo* and *in vitro* and, in addition, members of this genus produce large quantities of loose slime.

Cultural requirements

Similar to those of genera described above.

Cultural appearances
Non-capsulate, non-slime-forming mutants produce colonies similar to those of *Esch. coli* but normally the colonies are very viscid due to the extracellular materials which they produce.

Biochemical activities
These are not normally tested in diagnostic laboratories where identification is usually made on colonial appearances; urease is produced but *much more slowly* than by *Proteus* species and the lack of motility of *Klebsiellae* prevents confusion with Proteus organisms.

Serological characteristics
Somatic antigens in klebsiellae are usually masked by the capsular (K) antigens and/or the slime (M) antigens; in any one strain the M and K antigens are identical and by employing capsular antisera one can recognize at least 70 serotypes. The method of typing is the same as that used for pneumococci—the so-called capsule-swelling reaction.

Epidemiology
Although certain serotypes of *Klebsiella* are causally related to infections of the urinary tract and wounds and one particular species, *Kl. pneumoniae*, carries a high mortality rate on the infrequent occasions when it causes pneumonia, it must be appreciated that the majority are saprophytic or commensal.

Whilst *Klebsiella* strains are incriminated in urinary tract infections, they feature particularly in cases where there are predisposing gross lesions and are much less common where such lesions do not exist; infection may be endogenous or exogenous.

Apart from the occasional severe case of pneumonia, members of the genus are also found in some cases of paranasal sinusitis and acute otitis media, but it is not yet clear whether such organisms have been derived from an exogenous source or have existed as commensals in the upper respiratory tract prior to showing their pathogenic potential.

In addition to the genera mentioned above, there are several others in the family *Enterobacteriaceae*, e.g. *Cloaca, Hafnia*, but these are not considered here since they are rarely encountered as human pathogens, or perhaps one should say they are not recognized!

CHAPTER 19
Gram-negative bacilli, II

PSEUDOMONAS PYOCYANEA (*Ps. aeruginosa*)

Morphology
Size variable but approximately $1.5\mu m \times 0.5\mu m$, motile with polar flagella or often a single flagellum; non-capsulate, non-sporing.

Cultural requirements
Aerobic—most strains strictly so; wide temperature range for growth 5–43°C, optimum 37°C. Grows on ordinary media.

Cultural appearances
Colonies measure 2–4 mm and are low-convex, circular and often have an irregular spreading edge; cultures have a characteristic musty odour. Many strains produce pigments, pyocyanin and fluorescin, and their colonies have a greenish-blue fluorescent appearance. Some strains produce pyorubrin which endows their colonies with a reddish-brown colour. A significant minority of strains are unable to produce pigments even when special media are used for their detection. On MacConkey's medium colonies are similar in appearance but are pale since lactose is not fermented.

Heavily mucoid strains are occasionally isolated and almost invariably from the sputum of cases of cystic fibrosis.

Biochemical activities
With the exception of glucose none of the sugars usually employed in diagnostic laboratories is utilized. The oxidase test is positive within 30 sec of the reagent being applied to a culture of *Ps. pyocyanea*, and although a few other Gram-negative bacilli also react with the test

121

solution they do so much more slowly and rarely within 2 min. Thus the test is valuable in identifying strains which do not produce pigments.

Serological characteristics
Several attempts have been made to serotype strains on the basis of somatic and flagellar antigens but none of the schemes has been widely accepted. The epidemiological tracing of strains has been simplified by the introduction of type-identification by pyocine production—a method similar to that used in typing strains of *Sh. sonnei*.

Epidemiology of *Ps. pyocyanea* infections
Although there are more than 140 species in the genus *Pseudomonas* only *Ps. pyocyanea* is pathogenic to man; some other members are pathogenic for plants and animals but the majority lead a saprophytic existence.

Ps. pyocyanea also occurs widely in nature and is present as a commensal in the intestine of man and can be isolated from healthy skin. In fulfilling a pathogenic role it is often associated with pyogenic cocci or with one or other of the enterobacteria, e.g. *Esch. coli*, and its importance as a human pathogen has increased, particularly in the hospital environment since the introduction of antibiotics, to almost all of which it is naturally resistant.

Whilst infection may be endogenous, exogenous sources are other human cases and to a lesser extent carriers; methods of spread are probably mainly by indirect contact and via dust. The very wide temperature range for growth explains why *Pseudomonas* strains living in drains, mop-pails, sinks, etc., can multiply very easily so that the entire environment becomes contaminated. Similarly many pieces of apparatus in hospital, e.g. respirators, once contaminated, can act as vehicles of infection.

The ability of the organism to resist many disinfectants accounts for some hospital epidemics since a particular contaminated lotion or solution may be applied to many patients from a communal container.

Infection may be localized to a wound, burn, or to the urinary tract but in patients already debilitated, e.g. with multiple injuries, fatal septicaemias occur frequently.

Prevention
Prevention of exogenously acquired infection demands that patients who are suffering infection should be nursed in isolation and that patients who are particularly susceptible to infection should also be

nursed in strict isolation. Even so, the individual is at risk unless instruments, respirators, etc., are carefully and completely sterilized before use. With strict adherence to aseptic procedures the risk of infection will be reduced but even in isolation the ubiquitous nature of *Ps. pyocyanea* dictates the possibility of infection from fomites. Bacteriological monitoring of wards, etc., has revealed that even when all obvious vehicles have been eliminated bacilli can still be detected and may be present in the most mundane situations and transmitted to patients, e.g. strains will flourish in the earth of potted plants, and if the latter are watered by being left overnight in a partly filled bath, *Ps. pyocyanea* can be recovered from the bath after it has been emptied and cleaned!

BACTEROIDES

Morphology
The most commonly encountered species is *B. fragilis* which measures approximately $3\mu m \times 0.7\mu m$, non-motile, non-capsulate and non-sporing. Pleomorphism commonly encountered. *B. necrophorus* is a larger organism characteristically filamentous and with a weakly stained central bar but pleomorphism is marked.

Cultural requirements
Strictly anaerobic, wide temperate range, optimum 37°C. Incorporation of 20% bile in media enhances growth of all strains of *B. fragilis* whereas other species may be inhibited.

Cultural appearances
Growth is slow even under optimal conditions and on blood agar colonies are 1–2 mm in diameter after 48-hr incubation. Haemolysis is rarely encountered and colonies are circular, entire and convex with a smooth grey or greyish-white appearance.

Biochemical activities
B. fragilis can be differentiated from other species, e.g. *B. necrophorus* and *B. melaninogenicus* on the basis of varying patterns of sugar fermentation reactions.

Epidemiology of *Bacteroides* infections
Such species are commensal in the buccal cavity and the gastrointestinal tract and may also be isolated in healthy subjects from specimens of urine and the female genital tract. *B. fragilis* is the most common of all

commensal bacteria in the large bowel and like lactobacilli plays a role in protecting the gut against pathogenic species; however, unlike lactobacilli, bacteroides species can cause infections in various body tracts and tissues. Other bacteroides species include *B. necrophorus* which is commensal in the mouth and *B. melaninogenicus*; colonies of the latter commonly but not uniquely produce black pigmented colonies after incubation for 2–5 days on blood agar.

Bacteroides species are opportunistic pathogens and like *Ps. pyocyanea* often require the presence of precipitating factors, e.g. diabetes or the use of cytotoxic drugs before they display their pathogenicity. Infection is almost invariably endogenous in origin and although such infections are usually localized, bacteraemia is being increasingly recognized.

CHAPTER 20
Gram-negative bacilli, III

PARVOBACTERIA

The term parvobacteria is used to indicate a number of different bacterial genera which have some features in common; they are all small Gram-negative cocco-bacilli, may display pleomorphism. They are aerobes and usually with exacting requirements for growth.

HAEMOPHILI

H. INFLUENZAE

Morphology
Usually appear as small cocco-bacilli, only $1 \cdot 5 \mu m \times 0 \cdot 5 \mu m$, non-motile and non-sporing; capsulate in young cultures. In old cultures, and also in CSF from cases of meningitis caused by *H. influenzae*, the bacilli often appear as very long slender filaments.

Cultural requirements
Aerobic, temperature range for growth is 23–39°C, optimum 37°C. Will not grow on nutrient agar and requires both haematin (X factor) and nicotinamide-adenine dinucleotide (V factor) to be present before it will grow; these are supplied by incorporating blood in the medium.

Cultural appearances
On blood agar colonies are small (1 mm) and transparent with an entire edge. If the essential X and V factors are liberated from the blood cells in the agar plate by heating, thus producing what is known as a chocolate agar plate, growth is enhanced. Similarly, if grown in mixed culture with another species which produces V factor in abundance,

e.g. staphylococci, *H. influenzae* colonies, in the vicinity of colonies
of these other species, are much larger in size. This is known as *satellitism*.

Biochemical activities
Strains vary in their fermentative capacities and in any case their
activities are feeble.

Serological characteristics
Freshly isolated capsulate strains can be allocated to one of six serotypes (a–f) by noting, in capsule-swelling tests, which of six type-specific antisera reacts with the strain.

Epidemiology
H. influenzae is a strict parasite and man is the only host; both capsulate
and non-capsulate strains are found in the throats of healthy people.
Although the method of spread from person to person is not known, it
is probably by direct droplet spray since the organism is feebly viable
outside the host's tissues. As well as fulfilling a commensal role, *H. influenzae* can act as a secondary invader in the respiratory tract following
infection with other microorganisms. Influenza bacilli are commonly
found in chronic bronchitis and since clinical improvement follows
antimicrobial therapy which eliminates them they are assumed to participate in the disease process.

    H. influenzae is incriminated as a common cause of pyogenic meningitis, especially in children of pre-school age, and in this and other
infections serotype b strains are isolated more frequently than strains
of the five other types.

    Contrary to earlier suggestions, influenza bacilli are not causally related to influenza, although they may act as secondary invaders in this
and other virus infections of the respiratory tract.

Prevention
Only in people at special risk are any prophylactic steps taken. In those
suffering from chronic bronchitis long-term treatment with a tetracycline, particularly during the winter months, reduces the incidence
of acute bronchitic episodes.

OTHER HAEMOPHILI

H. aegyptius (Koch-Weeks bacillus) causes an acute, highly infectious
type of conjunctivitis; in its morphology, cultural requirements, etc., it

is very similar to *H. influenzae*. It can, however, be differentiated from the latter by serological tests.

H. ducreyii is the cause of chancroid, a venereal infection, and although similar in size to the influenza bacillus it frequently appears in pairs and short chains. It is extremely difficult to grow although it does not require the V factor.

H. haemolyticus deserves special mention since it occurs as a commensal in the throat and because of its colonial similarity to β-haemolytic streptococci may be confused with the latter; thus a false positive report may be given to the clinician. However, apart from their different reactions to Gram's strain, the application of a Bacitracin disk in the well of the inoculated culture plate easily prevents such errors since *H. haemolyticus* is resistant to this antibiotic whereas Group A β-haemolytic streptococci are sensitive.

BORDETELLAE

BORD. PERTUSSIS

Morphology
Similar to *H. influenzae*.

Cultural requirements
Very similar to *H. influenzae* but on subculture can be grown on ordinary media; for primary isolation, however, must be grown on Bordet-Gengou medium. Does not require X or V factors.

Cultural appearances
Growth may not be apparent until after 2–3 days incubation at 37°C. Colonies are minute, 1–2 mm in diameter with a circular edge and are dome-shaped and glistening and have been likened to a bisected pearl.

Biochemical activities
Devoid of fermentative powers.

Serological characteristics
All freshly isolated strains possess a common antigen, antigen 1, and may also have one or more of antigens 2, 3 and 4; thus fresh isolates can be typed. On subculture the antigenic structure becomes less distinct as isolates lose their pathogenicity.

Epidemiology of whooping cough
Infection is acquired from other *cases* of whooping cough and the fact that fresh cases occur without any known association with typical cases

does not imply that a carrier state exists; on the contrary, *Bord. pertussis* cannot be isolated from healthy individuals and infection can arise from cases which are not recognized as suffering from the disease either because the attack is naturally mild or has been modified by active immunization.

Bord. pertussis is most probably spread by direct droplet spray.

Whooping cough can occur at all ages but the incidence is greatest in pre-school children and the fact that a case is most infectious in the catarrhal stage of the illness, and before paroxysms allow a clinical diagnosis, probably explains its epidemic spread. Epidemics occur classically in regular cycles at two- or three-yearly intervals.

Prevention
Since the case is most infectious before the classical symptoms appear, isolation is relatively ineffective in preventing secondary cases if it is delayed until the patient is in the paroxysmal stage of the illness. A high degree of protection is afforded by active immunization as a potent vaccine will reduce the attack rate in home contacts of cases from approximately 90% in the unprotected siblings to less than 5% in contacts who have been fully immunized. Since nearly all deaths from whooping cough occur in the first year of life, immunization should begin as early as possible, i.e. between the 2nd and 6th month after birth.

OTHER *BORDETELLAE*

Bord. parapertussis is morphologically identical with *Bord. pertussis* but grows more rapidly on Bordet-Gengou medium and its colonies are very similar to those of the whooping cough bacillus but the underlying medium is discoloured by a brown pigment.

Parapertussis strains are serologically distinct and although they are occasionally associated with cases of whooping cough the illness is much less severe than that caused by *Bord. pertussis*.

PASTEURELLAE

P. PESTIS

Morphology
Short bacilli with rounded ends, $1 \cdot 5 \mu$m × $0 \cdot 7 \mu$m. Capsulate in the tissues and on first isolation in the laboratory; non-motile, non-sporing. Bipolar staining is characteristic and helpful in identification as, when methylene blue is applied, the poles of each bacillus stain more deeply than the central portion.

Cultural requirements
Aerobic and facultatively anaerobic. Temperature range for growth is 14–42°C with an *optimum of 27°C*, although subcultures will grow at 37°C; grows on ordinary media but growth is enhanced if blood is added to the medium.

Cultural appearances
Colonies are at first small (1 mm in diameter or less), transparent and with a circular edge; on continued incubation they may increase to 3–4 mm in diameter and have an irregular edge.

Biochemical activities
Glucose, mannitol and maltose are fermented without gas production and *P. pestis* will grow on MacConkey's medium in contrast to haemophili, bordetellae and other pasteurellae with the exception of *P. pseudotuberculosis*. However, unlike the plague bacillus, the latter is motile if tested at 22°C.

Serological characteristics
Strains are serologically homogeneous and also share certain antigens with other *Pasteurellae*.

Animal pathogenicity
Since plague is epizootic in wild rats it would be surprising if the causal organism did not affect rodents used in laboratory diagnostic procedures. If a white rat is injected subcutaneously with a freshly isolated strain of *P. pestis* it dies in 2–3 days; post-mortem examination reveals a necrotic lesion at the point of injection and the regional lymph glands are also involved. In addition to these sites the bacilli can also be recovered from the heart blood and from the enlarged spleen.

Epidemiology of plague
Plague is primarily a disease of rats and other rodents and man is only involved as a secondary host under certain environmental circumstances. In the past, human epidemics were greatly feared and rightly so; for example, in the Black Death of the 14th century, it has been estimated that at least 25% of the population of Europe died.

The bacilli are spread from the rodent host by rat fleas such as *Xenopsylla cheopis*; the flea takes a blood meal from the infected rodent and the bacilli multiply in its stomach and proventriculus, which becomes blocked. If the flea alights on a new host and attempts another blood meal, regurgitation from the blocked proventriculus ensures that plague bacilli are inoculated into the bite wound.

In man there follows an incubation period 3–7 days before the related lymph glands show evidence of infection; these swell and the surrounding tissues become oedematous so that a primary bubo is formed. In *bubonic* plague secondary buboes may develop along the lymphatic system and if the organisms spread into the blood stream the patient dies from septicaemic plague. Some cases are primarily septicaemic and death may occur before buboes develop fully.

In bubonic plague, infection rarely spreads to other men and fresh cases in an epidemic are individually infected by rat fleas. If, however, pulmonary infection results during a septicaemic phase the patient may act as a source from which other people may acquire *pneumonic plague* either from dust particles contaminated from the sputum or by infected droplets.

Prevention

Rodent control is vitally important, particularly to prevent their importation by a ship or plane whose voyage started from a country where plague occurs. Various vaccines are available but the degree of protection which they give is variable, particularly that made from dead bacilli, e.g. Haffkine's vaccine.

Patients must be treated in isolation and when an epidemic begins intensive flea control should be undertaken as well as rat control. Personnel working in the epidemic area should wear protective clothing which is dusted regularly with insecticide and in addition insect repellant cream should be used. Prophylactic dosing with tetracyclines has been recommended for medical and nursing personnel dealing with cases.

OTHER *PASTEURELLAE*

Only a few of the other members of the genus *Pasteurella* are pathogenic to man and they are rarely encountered; they do, however, cause infection in many animals and birds. Other species are morphologically indistinguishable from *P. pestis* but can be differentiated from it and from each other by biochemical means and also by their varying virulence to different animals.

P. septica is not only carried by several domestic animals and poultry but can cause disease in the natural host. Wounds in man inflicted by the bites of dogs or cats may be infected with such strains which apparently delay healing of the wound.

P. haemolytica may be carried by healthy cattle and sheep but occasionally causes pneumonia in these animals; non-pathogenic to man.

P. pseudotuberculosis causes a tuberculosis-like disease in several animals including guinea-pigs. It may do this in laboratory guinea-pigs, and so confuse the bacteriologist performing necropsy on animals infected by it which have been injected with pathological material from a suspect human case of tuberculosis.

P. pseudotuberculosis is not acid-fast so that although the lesions it causes may resemble those of tuberculosis, a Z-N stained film of material from them rapidly resolves any doubt as to the nature of the causal organism. *P. pseudotuberculosis* differs from other members of the genus in being motile when grown at 22°C and, like *P. pestis*, growth occurs on MacConkey's medium but growth is more abundant and more rapid than that of the plague bacillus.

BRUCELLAE

BR. ABORTUS

Morphology

Small cocco-bacilli and frequently almost coccal in appearance; approximately 0·4μm–0·6μm. Rarely capsulate; non-motile and non-sporing.

Cultural requirements

Aerobic but requires presence of 5–10% CO_2 for primary isolation. Will grow on ordinary media, but growth is accelerated and enhanced if the medium contains animal protein, e.g. on liver-infusion agar. Temperature range for growth is 20–40°C. Optimum is 37°C.

Cultural appearances

Growth is slow even under optimal conditions; colonies are small, low-convex and with an entire edge. On continued incubation they increase in size and their original translucence is lost and they become yellowish and eventually brown.

Biochemical activities

No fermentative properties unless the carbohydrate substrates are incorporated in a peptone-free, buffered medium; under these conditions *Br. abortus* can be differentiated from the two other members of the genus since it utilizes glucose and inositol.

More commonly, such differentiation is carried out by checking the

ability of strains to grow in the presence of 1 in 25 000 basic fuchsin
and 1 in 30 000 thionine; *Br. abortus* is inhibited by thionine.

Serological characteristics
In common with the other members of the genus, *Br. abortus* possesses
two antigens, A (abortus) and M (melitensis); however, although antiserum prepared against *Br. abortus* contains both A and M antibodies
the latter type can be removed by absorption with a suspension of
Br. melitensis and the absorbed serum then reacts only with *Br. abortus*.
The preparation of such absorbed antisera is possible since M antigen
predominates in *Br. melitensis* and its relatively poor content of A
antigen does not significantly alter the level of A antibody in the serum
during absorption.

Animal pathogenicity
Guinea-pigs are susceptible to experimental infection but are not
normally used for diagnostic purposes; other experimental animals are
less susceptible.

Epidemiology of brucellosis
Br. abortus occurs naturally in cattle and is responsible for epidemics
of abortion in such animals. *Br. melitensis* is primarily pathogenic for
goats and sheep whilst *Br. suis* occurs in pigs. These host specificities
are not abolute and man is susceptible to infection by all three species.
Infection in man can occur in two ways: *first* by consumption of milk
and freshly prepared milk products, such as cheese and butter made
from infected milk, and *secondly* the organisms can enter via skin
abrasions.

In Britain, *Br. abortus* is the species most commonly encountered in
human cases and it is interesting that abortion is very rare in women
who suffer brucellosis. It is considered that this is because human
placentae do not contain *erythritol*, which abounds in the placental
tissues of cows, sheep and goats. This is known to stimulate the growth
of brucellae and the subsequent placentitis causes abortion.

Brucellosis also occurs as an occupational infection in farmers,
veterinary surgeons and butchers. The organisms enter through skin
abrasions when the individual is handling infected discharges or
carcases.

Prevention
Pasteurization of milk protects the general population against this
source of infection; abortion in cattle has been reduced by widespread

vaccination but abortus infection is still endemic and the need for pasteurization before milk is consumed has not declined.

A government-sponsored Brucellosis Eradication scheme is now being undertaken in Britain with the aim of creating cattle herds free from this infection; the scheme is analogous to that which eradicated tuberculosis in our cattle and hopefully should be as successful.

Those following occupations which have a risk of infection must be educated in the handling and disposal of infected excreta, dead foetuses and other infected carcases. There is no vaccine available for human use.

OTHER *BRUCELLAE*

Br. melitensis and *Br. suis* are morphologically identical with *Br. abortus* and their cultural requirements differ only in that they do not require increased CO_2 in their atmosphere for primary isolation. Their colonial appearances do not differ from those of *Br. abortus* but they are differentiated by sensitivity to dyes; *Br. melitensis* is not inhibited either by basic fuchsin or thionine, whereas *Br. suis* is inhibited by basic fuchsin. Similarly *Br. melitensis* does not produce H_2S and members of the other two species do so; *Br. suis* strains from American sources differ from Danish strains only in their ability to produce H_2S.

CHAPTER 21
Vibrios and Spirilla

VIBRIO CHOLERAE

Morphology
Often termed the comma bacillus on account of its curved shape, approximately $2–3\mu m \times 0·5\mu m$, Gram-negative, motile by virtue of a single terminal flagellum, non-capsulate, non-sporing. Characteristic shape usually lost on *in vitro* cultivation.

Cultural requirements
Aerobic, temperature range for growth 16–40°C, optimum 37°C. Sensitive to acid pH, thus media must be adjusted accordingly; optimum pH 8·2.

Cultural appearances
Colonies are not distinctive and are variable; a 'typical' colony is large, 2–3 mm in diameter after overnight incubation at 37°C, with an entire edge and is translucent. Older colonies may develop a yellowish colour.

Biochemical activities
Ferments a variety of sugars without production of gas. Gives a positive *cholera-red reaction*, i.e. when grown in peptone water, cholera vibrios produce indole and nitrites so that when a few drops of H_2SO_4 are added to an overnight culture a pink colour develops due to the production of the red compound nitroso-indole.

Does not cause haemolysis when 1 ml of a 48-hr broth culture is added to an equal volume of a 5% suspension of sheep RBC; this is known as the Greig test.

Serological characteristics
Cholera vibrios are serologically homogeneous in regard to their
flagellar and major somatic antigens; however, minor somatic antigens
allow the differentiation of two serotypes 'Inaba' and 'Ogawa'.

Epidemiology of cholera
Although an individual recovering from cholera may be a temporary
carrier for one or two weeks, chronic carriage beyond this period is
exceptional; thus *cases* of the disease are the main source of infection.
Man is the only host. The main method of epidemic spread is by water
supplies contaminated by cases and the temperature growth range
allows the vibrios to multiply in water tanks so that explosive outbreaks
are commonly seen; case to case infection via contaminated foodstuffs
also occurs and insanitary methods of disposing of excreta may allow
insects to contaminate food.

The emergence of the El Tor biotype of *V. cholerae* in Indonesia in
1961 heralded a pandemic spread of cholera and within ten years this
species invaded the Far East and then spread to India, Pakistan, the
Middle East and Southern Russia before establishing itself in many
African countries and Spain; importations to several European countries have occurred recently. Although contaminated water supplies are
also incriminated in the spread of cholera due to the El Tor vibrio,
carriage of the latter is more frequent and more persistent than of
V. cholerae so that direct person-to-person spread of the former is a
greater hazard than in infections caused by *V. cholerae*.

Prevention
In the past cholera occurred pandemically and visited Europe and North
America in epidemic waves even in the latter half of the last century;
its elimination from many countries was due primarily to the creation
of water supply systems which, in addition to incorporating physical
and chemical purification techniques, also eliminated the possibility of
the water being contaminated by man after purification had taken place.
In countries where safe water supplies are not yet available emergency
treatment, with hypochlorite, of bulk supplies in storage tanks is
practicable and, in any case, water for human consumption or for use
in food preparation must be boiled.

Obviously cases of the disease should be treated in isolation and apart
from combating the fluid and electrolyte imbalance caused by the
profuse diarrhoea which would otherwise kill the patient, the administration of a suitable antibiotic will eliminate the vibrios and shorten

the period in which the convalescent is a risk to the community.

Cholera vaccine given in two doses at 7-day intervals may give some degree of protection for a month or two but its real value is not known.

OTHER VIBRIOS

The El Tor vibrio has many similarities to *V. cholerae* and infections caused by El Tor vibrios are clinically indistinguishable from those caused by the classical strains.

It can be distinguished from *V. cholerae* in giving a positive Greig test, by its ability to cause haemagglutination of fowl RBC and by its resistance to polymyxin B. In addition, El Tor strains are resistant to the activity of phages which lyse *V. cholerae*.

Many other vibrios can be identified and several are causally related to diseases in various animals; others are saprophytic in water.

SPIRILLUM MINUS

Morphology

$2–5\mu m \times 0.5\mu m$, rigid spiralled organism; Gram-negative and actively motile with bipolar lophotrichous flagella. Non-capsulate and non-sporing.

This organism, which is the only member of the genus *Spirillum* known to be pathogenic to man has not been successfully cultured *in vitro* and hence its other biological characteristics are unknown.

Sp. minus is a natural parasite of rats, mice and other rodents and man may suffer infection if bitten by an infected rodent. In cases of rat-bite fever the organism can be demonstrated in material from the bite wound, the regional lymph glands and on occasion in the blood either by microscopy or by intraperitoneal inoculation of material into a guinea-pig. The animal develops a chronic febrile illness and spirilla can be detected in its blood and also in the lymph glands 7–14 days after inoculation; at post-mortem the organism can be demonstrated in most tissues and organs.

Cases of rat-bite fever are sporadic and preventive measures are obvious.

CHAPTER 22
Spirochaetes

1 BORRELIAE

BORR. VINCENTII

Morphology
5–20μm × 0·4μm, with 3–8 coils which are irregular in amplitude; Gram-negative, non-capsulate, non-sporing.

Cultural requirements
Strictly anaerobic and very difficult to grow in pure culture; cultivation is never attempted for diagnostic purposes.

Borr. vincentii is found in *small* numbers in the healthy human mouth and in association with a large, cigar-shaped, bacillus *Fusobacterium fusiforme*. In mouths in a poor state of dental hygiene and particularly when the individual is suffering other buccal infection or is malnourished, e.g. suffering from Vitamin C deficiency, very much larger numbers of these two organisms can be detected, particularly in films made from the lesions of Vincent's infection. There is doubt as to whether the symbionts are primarily responsible for the infection but since it responds to penicillin quite dramatically there is no doubt that they have a causal role, perhaps as secondary pathogens.

The disease is, therefore, endogenous and usually sporadic, but occasional epidemics have been reported; prevention depends on maintenance of oral hygiene and correction of any nutritional deficiencies.

OTHER *BORRELIAE*

Other members of the genus cause diseases in domestic animals and poultry and some occur as commensals of man; however, one or two are incriminated as the causal agents of relapsing fever and are transmitted from case to case by lice or ticks.

Borr. recurrentis, the causal organism of European relapsing fever, is similar in morphological appearance to *Borr. vincentii* except that the coils have a regular amplitude. It can be harvested in a variety of fluid media under anaerobic conditions but diagnosis usually involves only the demonstration of the organism in films of peripheral blood or by injecting white rats with a blood sample from the patient. The organism is transmitted from case to case by the body louse which infects a bite-wound with its excreta; alternatively, lice may be crushed when the individual scratches, thus inoculating himself through skin abrasions.

Borr. duttonii is identical with *Borr. recurrentis* with the exception of its distinctive antigenic make-up; it causes West African relapsing fever and is tick-borne. Spread of infection may be from case to case via the tick or may be transmitted by the tick to man from primary hosts, e.g. rodents and pigs. A tick may remain infected for some years after having a blood meal and spirochaetes are also transmitted transovarially to consecutive generations of ticks.

Several other borreliae have been incriminated as causing relapsing fever in other countries and on insufficient evidence have been given species designation.

2 TREPONEMATA

TR. PALLIDUM

Morphology

6–14μm × 0·1μm, and possessing 6–12 regular coils. So fine is the spiral filament that it cannot be seen in film preparations stained by ordinary methods; the organisms can be seen by dark-ground illumination or, alternatively, by the ordinary light microscope after their size has been increased by silver impregnation staining.

Tr. pallidum has not been grown *in vitro* and hence we know nothing of its biochemical or other characteristics; nevertheless, in syphilitic patients antibodies can be detected which immobilize *Tr. pallidum* strains maintained in the laboratory by intratesticular inoculation of rabbits. Such antibodies can also fix complement but in these tests the stock antigen is an extract from normal tissues and does not contain *Tr. pallidum*.

Epidemiology of syphilis

Sources are cases in the primary and secondary stages of the illness and with few exceptions infection is contracted during sexual intercourse; exceptions to this rule include acquisition of a primary lesion on the hand of the unsuspecting medical practitioner. *Tr. pallidum* dies so rapidly outside the host tissues that transfer by indirect contact is extremely rare.

Congenital syphilis, i.e. intrauterine infection of the foetus via the placenta, is very much less common nowadays and this reduction in incidence reflects the dramatic advances in antenatal care which have occurred in the last 30 years and also the efficiency of antibiotics in treating adult cases.

Prevention

Since a single source gives rise to several new cases, sometimes as many as 30 or more, prevention demands speedy diagnosis and treatment to render the patient non-infectious as rapidly as possible and, simultaneously, the tracing of contacts of each new case must be rigorous. Whilst in some countries compulsory powers are used to trace contacts, prevent default from treatment, etc., in Britain the voluntary system of control is preferred in combination with health and sex education.

OTHER *TREPONEMATA*

Many organisms resembling *Tr. pallidum* occur commensally in man and some of these are resident on the genital mucosa and might confuse the diagnosis when a suspected case of primary syphilis is being investigated; however, if care is taken to thoroughly clean the area before collecting exudate from the lesion, commensals such as *Tr. gracile* will not be collected in the specimen.

Although *Tr. pallidum* is the only pathogenic member of the genus found in Britain, other treponematoses occur but almost entirely in tropical countries. None of these is sexually acquired and infection is probably transmitted by personal contact or by drinking from contaminated communal cups as is the case with *bejel*, which is essentially a disease of children, and which presents with lesions similar to those of secondary syphilis without a primary lesion having occurred.

Another non-venereal infection which is better known than bejel is *yaws*, where transmission of the causal organism, *Tr. pertenue*, is by direct contact or by flies which feed on lesions. Organisms which survive in the proventriculus for several hours are regurgitated when the fly has another feed. *Tr. pertenue* is biologically identical with *Tr. pallidum*.

Tr. carateum is responsible for the disease *pinta* which occurs particularly in South American countries; this organism is indistinguishable from that causing syphilis but it is likely that they differ in antigenic constitution since individuals suffering from syphilis can acquire pinta and vice versa.

3 LEPTOSPIRAE

L. ICTEROHAEMORRHAGIAE

Morphology

6–20μm × 0·1μm, coils are very numerous, small and close together and although visible with dark-ground illumination they are obscured if stained preparations are examined; one or both ends of the organism are recurved on the body.

Cultural requirements

Unlike members of the genera *Borrelia* and *Treponema*, leptospirae can be isolated *in vitro* for diagnostic purposes and although solid media are available for research purposes the organism grows more readily in fluid media, e.g. Stuart's, provided these contain animal serum. Essentially microaerophilic and with an optimum temperature of 30°C. Sensitive to acid environments.

Biochemical activities

No knowledge available.

Serological characteristics

Certain antigens are shared with some other pathogenic leptospirae, but antigens specific for *L. icterohaemorrhagiae* allow us to prepare antiserum which can be absorbed by leptospirae possessing only the shared antigens. Such absorbed antiserum can them be employed in agglutination tests to identify newly isolated strains. Because of the morphological similarity of all leptospirae and our inability to use cultural or biochemical methods of establishing the separate identities of various strains, we rely entirely on serological methods of identification.

Animal pathogenicity

Young guinea-pigs and golden hamsters are most susceptible and after intraperitoneal inoculation with pathological material containing leptospirae, e.g. patient's blood, or with freshly isolated laboratory cultures, the animal shows progressive fever and then jaundice and dies in 10–14 days. At post-mortem there is generalized jaundice and hae-morrhage, the spleen and adrenals are enlarged and friable and the spirochaetes can be recovered from many organs and are most numer-ous in the liver.

Epidemiology of Weil's disease

Weil's disease is the name given to human infection caused by *L. ictero-haemorrhagiae*. This organism lives normally in the brown rat and there leads an essentially commensal existence and is localized in the rat's kidneys and is thus discharged in the urine. Organisms discharged into man's environment may survive for only an hour or two unless they are in moist surroundings with an alkaline pH; thus, in Britain, Weil's disease is to a large extent associated with certain occupations such as mining, fish-gutting, etc., where people are working in damp, rat-infested places.

The organisms penetrate through cuts and abrasions in skin and mucous membranes and occasional cases arise through people bathing in canals, rivers or stagnant ponds which are populated by rats. Like almost all other zoonoses, Weil's disease does not spread from patients to other human beings.

Prevention

Individuals engaged in high-risk ocupations must be taught about sources of infection and the methods of its spread, and wherever pos-sible should wear protective clothing; eradication of rats, and rodent proofing, should be undertaken.

Washing down of working surfaces, e.g. slabs in fish-gutting halls, with acid solutions also assists protection of workers.

OTHER PATHOGENIC *LEPTOSPIRAE*

Numerous serotypes have been identified throughout the world and these are frequently associated with various natural hosts; apart from *L. icterohaemorrhagiae* only one other type, *L. canicola*, occurs in Britain. The resultant illness in man is Canicola fever which is much milder than Weil's disease, frequently anicteric and rarely fatal. Dogs and pigs act as natural hosts and man becomes infected by mopping up dog's urine or by working in piggeries.

It should be noted that the genus *Leptospira* is subject to the con-tinuing epidemic of change in bacterial nomenclature and that all pathogenic leptospirae are entitled *Leptospira interrogans* and serotypes are defined, e.g. *L. interrogans* serotype *icterohaemorrhagiae*.

Similarly saprophytic strains within the genus are now collectively named *L. biflexa*.

Whilst this and other examples of taxonomic correctness may be welcomed by the purist, there is an increasing danger that such changes, if rapidly introduced in reporting results to clinicians, may cause a breakdown in the communication system which is already tenuous.

CHAPTER 23
Higher bacteria

Within the higher bacteria two families, *Streptomycetaceae* and *Actinomycetaceae*, have medical significance. In the former family some members of the genus *Streptomyces* produce clinically useful antibiotics, such as streptomycin from *Streptomyces griseus*.

Higher bacteria pathogenic to man and animals belong to the *Actinomycetaceae* and here two genera, *Actinomyces* and *Nocardia* must be considered.

1 ACTINOMYCES

ACTINO. ISRAELII

Morphology
Branching filaments approximately 1μm in diameter which interlace to form a mycelium. Gram-positive, non-motile, non-capsulate, non-sporing. Fragmentation of the filaments gives rise to bacillary and coccal forms. In sections of actinomycotic lesions stained by Gram's method, club-shaped structures which stain Gram-negatively can be noted at the periphery of the Gram-positive mycelium. A similar section stained by Ziehl-Neelsen's technique shows that these peripheral clubs are acid-fast if 1% H_2SO_4 is used in attempted decolourization instead of a 20% solution as for *M. tuberculosis*.

Cultural requirements
Anaerobic or microaerophilic atmosphere is required; optimum temperature for growth is 37°C and growth does not take place at temperatures much above or below the optimum; grows on ordinary agar but greatly enhanced if serum or blood is incorporated.

Cultural appearances
Colonies show considerable variation but are nodular, opaque and
ochre in colour so called 'bread crumb type' colonies; firmly adherent
to underlying medium.

Biochemical activities
These are saccharolytic but there is much variation among strains and
thus no reliance can be placed on such reactions.

Serological characteristics
Antigenic analysis permits the recognition of four serotypes of *Actino.
israelii* but at present such serotyping is essentially of academic importance.

Animal pathogenicity
Experimental inoculation of rabbits and guinea-pigs may or may not
result in nodular granulomatous lesions hence such methods are not
used in diagnosis.

Epidemiology of actinomycosis
Infection is endogenous from organisms which normally fulfil a commensal role in the mouth. Almost three-quarters of all lesions occur in
the oro-facial region and the disease is apparently precipitated by trauma
since there is frequently a history of, for example, dental extraction or,
in the case of abdominal actinomycosis, recent appendectomy or external trauma.

   In Britain actinomycosis is most prevalent among male agricultural
workers and it was once thought that the human disease was acquired
from cattle whose mouths in health often contain *Actino. bovis*. As well
as this commensal existence, this organism can produce a disease,
lumpy jaw, the bovine counterpart of human actinomycosis. In addition to its high incidence in agricultural workers actinomycosis is
much more common in men than in women (4 : 1) and the majority of
cases occur in the age group 10–29 years.

OTHER *ACTINOMYCES*

Actino. bovis is morphologically identical with *Actino. israelii* but it can
grow aerobically. Colonies are smoother than those of *Actino. israelii*
and do not adhere to the medium; biochemical activity is variable from

strain to strain but unlike *Actino. israelii*, *Actino. bovis* strains hydrolyse starch. Serologically unrelated to *Actino. israelii types*.

2 NOCARDIA

NOC. MADURAE

Morphology
Basically similar to *Actino. israelii* but filaments are narrower, i.e. 0·5μm. Acid-fastness is not a feature of *Noc. madurae*.

Cultural requirements
Obligate aerobe with an optimum growth temperature of 37°C. Grows on a wide range of media.

Cultural appearances
Like *Actino. israelii*, colonies are very adherent to the surface of the medium. On agar, colonies are at first small, round and convex but later they increase in size and become opaque with a rosette appearance. They are difficult to emulsify.

Biochemical activities
Has no saccharolytic powers.

Serological characteristics
Knowledge of antigenic structure is incomplete.

Noc. madurae is one of the causes of madura foot, a granulomatous infection confined to the feet which occurs only in the tropics and some sub-tropical countries. In addition to other nocardiae some cases of madura foot are caused by true fungi, e.g. *Madurella*.

There are more than 40 other members of the genus *Nocardia* but the majority of these are saprophytic; however, at least one other species, *Nocardia asteroides*, is pathogenic for man and in Britain this organism is responsible for pulmonary nocardial infection. Morphologically similar to *Noc. madurae*, it is *acid-fast*, a strict aerobe and its colonies are *star-shaped*. It produces acid from glucose.

CHAPTER 24
Specimens: Collection, delivery and processing

This section gives a synopsis of the methods of collection, delivery and the laboratory processing of the more commonly encountered specimens submitted for bacteriological examination; it is not comprehensive.

Unsatisfactory specimens are still submitted to laboratories but perhaps less frequently than in the past; this improvement reflects a greater awareness on the part of the clinician of the very obvious fact that no matter how scientific modern laboratory procedures may be, they cannot compensate for certain basic errors in the collection and transmission of specimens.

Special requirements for the various types of specimen are given in this chapter, but firstly some general points must be emphasized which, although glaringly obvious, are ignored from time to time.

1 All specimens must be accompanied with details of the patient's name, sex, age and address and the nature of the specimen; these are *minimal* requirements solely for the purposes of identification. Similarly, the doctor who submits the specimen should give his identity and address; in every laboratory there is a 'lost lambs' file containing request forms which may be completely blank or with insufficient information to allow identification of the patient and/or doctor. Each of these forms is not only a source of frustration to the laboratory staff but on occasion the patient's health or even life may be endangered and sometimes the community is placed at unnecessary risk, e.g. a specimen of faeces from an unknown source may be found to contain typhoid bacilli.

Additional information which should accompany the specimen includes the clinical diagnosis, duration of the illness, information regarding the patient's immune state, e.g. if previously immunized with TAB when serum is submitted for Widal testing, and whether antimicrobial therapy has been given.

146

2   No antiseptics or other antimicrobial agents should come into contact with the specimen; all specimen containers should be sterile before use and they can be supplied in this state by the laboratory.

3   In collecting the specimen care must be taken to avoid contamination of the outside of the container otherwise the clinician, the person delivering the specimen to the laboratory, and the laboratory staff may be infected.

4   Transmission of the specimen to the laboratory should be within a few hours; limits for certain types of specimen are specified under the individual headings.

5   If specimens are delivered by postal service certain regulations must be observed and these are known to the investigating laboratory which can provide suitable containers for this purpose. The important points in the regulations are:

(a) the specimen container should be sealed in such a way as to prevent the escape of pathological material and it must be placed in a suitable case which is padded with absorbent material;

(b) suitable cases are prescribed and are made either from wood or leatherboard;

(c) the outer envelope must be clearly marked 'Pathological Specimen' and 'Fragile with Care'; specimens can only be sent by letter post and not by parcel post.

BLOOD CULTURE

Certain basic facts must be stressed regarding the collection of venous blood for the attempted isolation of pathogens. Firstly as venepuncture is required it is essential that a fully aseptic technique is followed so that *the patient is not infected as a result of the diagnostic procedure.* Similarly extraneous contamination of the specimen must be avoided otherwise the laboratory may issue a misleading report. Since the bacterial population of the blood in bacteraemia may be very small, e.g. only one or two organisms per ml, at least 5 ml of blood should be collected. The laboratory can supply a variety of media for blood culture and each has its advantage in isolating particular pathogens so that the clinician who suspects that a patient is suffering from a particular infection should consult the bacteriologist concerning which media are most suited to the particular case.

It is important that the bacteriologist should be informed of any antibacterial therapy which the patient is receiving since he can then incorporate in the medium certain enzymes which will eliminate the continued activity of the antibacterial agent in the blood once it has been introduced to the culture medium. For example, penicillinase can be added to the broth if the patient has been receiving penicillin and this enhances the prospects of isolating any organisms present in the specimen; of course since only 5 ml of blood are added to 50 ml of broth any antibiotic present will be significantly diluted.

Delivery to the laboratory
Once inoculated, the blood culture bottle must be returned to the laboratory immediately and if this is not possible it must be maintained at a temperature as near as possible to, but not exceeding, 37°C.

Laboratory procedure
After 18–24 hr incubation at 37°C the blood-broth mixture is sampled by removing aseptically two or three loopfulls which are plated on to two blood agar plates, one of which is incubated at 37°C under aerobic conditions whilst the other is incubated anaerobically. Such sampling is repeated every 48 hr for at least 2–3 weeks before a negative report is issued; any organisms which are isolated are of course subjected to complete identification.

When the patient is suspected to be suffering from brucellosis a special blood culture bottle is used. This has a layer of liver-infusion agar lying along one side (in addition to the broth) and after delivery to the laboratory CO_2 is introduced to give a 5–10% concentration and the bottle is then incubated. The agar surface is inoculated by carefully tilting the bottle so that the blood-broth mixture flows gently over the medium; thus the bottle need not be opened every 48 hr for sampling and any brucellae present, particularly *Br. abortus*, will have optimal conditions for growth. Although colonies will usually be visible within 7 days the blood culture bottle should be incubated for 4 weeks before a negative report is issued in those instances when there is no growth.

CLOT CULTURE

In suspect cases of enteric fever the chances of isolating *S. typhi* or one of the paratyphoid bacilli during the bacteraemic phase of the illness are enhanced if clot culture is used instead of blood culture, even if a bile-salt broth is used in the latter method.

5 ml of venous blood are obtained by venepuncture and transferred into a suitable sterile container, e.g. a 2 oz screwcapped bottle, and allowed to clot. The serum is then removed aseptically and the clot is

lyzed by adding to it 15 ml of 0·5% bile-salt broth containing 1500 units of streptokinase. Thereafter the mixture is incubated at 37°C and examined every 48 hr in the same way as for blood culture. Not only is the isolation of salmonellae more frequently made by clot culture but there are also additional advantages; the clinician does not require a supply of special blood culture bottles and a Widal test can be carried out on the separated serum so that the titre obtained at this stage can be used as a base-line for the results of Widal tests later in the illness.

CEREBROSPINAL FLUID

The comments regarding the patient's safety and the prevention of contamination of the specimen made under 'blood culture' are equally pertinent in performing a lumbar puncture to obtain a specimen of cerebrospinal fluid (CSF).

Delivery to the laboratory
Delivery must be very rapid and the fluid should be warm when it arrives; if this is impossible then the container must be held at 37°C and in any case *not more than 4 hr should elapse* before laboratory processing is undertaken. This time and temperature requirement is dictated by the feeble powers of survival of some of the organisms which may cause meningitis, in particular the meningococcus and *H. influenzae*.

Laboratory procedure
1 *Macroscopic examination* of the specimen should be made for colour, turbidity and for the presence of any deposit or clot; then 1 ml of CSF is transferred aseptically to a tube containing a similar volume of 0·2% glucose broth which is then incubated for 24 hr at 37°C. The broth enhances the growth of meningococci and pneumococci if either of these species is present and subculture of the CSF-broth mixture, after incubation, is made to two blood agar plates, one of which is incubated aerobically and the other in an atmosphere containing 5% CO_2.

2 *A white cell count* is performed and the remaining CSF is then centrifuged at 3000 rev/min for 5 min; the supernatant is removed aseptically and sent for biochemical examination.

3 *The centrifuged deposit* is then used to make films which are stained by Gram's method and the deposit is also used to inoculate two blood agar plates which are incubated under the same conditions as the subcultures from the CSF-broth mixture as above.

4 CSF from *cases of tuberculous meningitis* frequently contain a 'spider-web' clot if the container is allowed to stand upright without being disturbed for 1–2 hr at 37°C and if a film is made with part of the clot and stained by the Ziehl-Neelsen method, tubercle bacilli may be seen.

In addition to microscopic examination of the clot, or alternatively if no clot is present, the CSF is centrifuged and the deposit is used to inoculate tubes of Lowenstein-Jensen medium and is also injected into a pair of guinea-pigs. Animal inoculation yields a higher proportion of positive results than does cultivation of the same specimen.

URINE

Although *mid-stream specimens* of urine from male patients have always been accepted as satisfactory for bacteriological examination, it is only in the last few years that there has been general agreement that such specimens from female patients are also reliable; in both sexes, provided that the patients are properly instructed, contamination of the urine can be avoided and the bacteriological results obtained with mid-stream specimens are as reliable as those with catheter specimens of urine.

Catheterization must be avoided wherever possible since *the procedure carries a definite risk of introducing infection.*

In the male the foreskin is retracted, the glans washed with soap and water and after voiding a little urine to flush commensal organisms, e.g. staphylococci and diphtheroids, from the anterior uretha the mid-flow of urine is collected in a suitable sterile screw-capped container; in women the ano-genital region is thoroughly washed and then with the labia widely separated the mid-stream urine is collected in a sterile wide-mouthed container, e.g. a 12 oz honey-pot.

Delivery to the laboratory
Since urine is an excellent culture medium the specimen must be transported to the laboratory within 1–2 hr otherwise any organisms present in the specimen will multiply and the results of quantitative examination will be misleading; if this time limit cannot be met the specimen must be stored in a refrigerator until collected or alternatively it may be delivered in a special container which maintains a low temperature.

Laboratory procedure
1 *Microscopic examination.* 5 ml of the specimen is centrifuged at 3000 rev/min for 5 min and the deposit resuspended in a small amount of

the supernatant after the larger part of the latter has been decanted. A wet film is made from the resuspended deposit and examined for the presence of bacteria, pus cells and red blood cells.

2 *Cultivation*. The resuspended deposit is also used to inoculate a blood agar plate and a plate of MacConkey's medium and if on microscopic examination any bacteria are present a primary sensitivity plate should also be seeded with the deposit. These plates are incubated overnight at 37°C and species identification is then made and, if necessary, subculture sensitivity tests are performed.

3 *Bacterial count*. Provided that the specimen is properly collected and is delivered to the laboratory within the conditions mentioned above then an estimation of the number of bacteria per ml of urine is valuable in deciding whether the bacterial population of the specimen is from established infection or has resulted merely from contamination. Separate dilutions of urine, 1 in 100 and 1 in 1000, are made in nutrient broth and then a known volume of each, e.g. 0·1 ml, is spread over the surface of two nutrient agar plates which are then incubated for 18–24 hr at 37°C. The colonies are then counted and assuming that each colony represents one organism in the original inoculum the number of bacteria per ml can be estimated.

Counts of 10^3 organisms or less per ml almost invariably reflect a contaminated specimen whereas if 10^5 or more organisms are found to be present in 1 ml this is indicative of infection. Counts in the region of 10^4 bacteria per ml may result either from contamination or infection and in such cases the count should be repeated on a fresh specimen; such counts probably result from contamination if more than one bacterial species is present.

Urinary tuberculosis

In cases suspected of suffering from tuberculous infection of the urinary tract the specimen submitted to the laboratory should be three consecutive early morning specimens which are pooled in the laboratory before examination.

Contamination of such specimens with commensal acid-fast *M. smegmatis* can be reduced by thorough washing of the genitalia before urine is passed.

Before such specimens can be examined they must be processed to reduce their volume, to kill organisms other than tubercle bacilli and to liquefy mucus or cells within which tubercle bacilli may be trapped. This processing is known as concentration and several methods are available but all make use of the relative resistance of tubercle bacilli to acids, alkalis or other mucolytic agents.

After concentration a film is made and stained by the Ziehl-Neelsen method and the concentrate is also used to inoculate slopes of Lowenstein-Jensen's medium and two guinea-pigs.

THROAT SWABS

It is essential that the throat should be examined and swabbed under adequate illumination; a spatula must be used to depress the tongue and the use of the handle of a domestic spoon or fork in place of a spatula must be condemned. Such narrow 'spatulae' only serve to force the edges of the tongue upwards and thus obscure a view of the tonsillar areas; if antiseptic lozenges have been sucked or if the patient has gargled then swabbing should be deferred for at least six hours.

Delivery to the laboratory
Swabs should be processed in the laboratory within 12 hr of being taken; some types of cotton-wool have a lethal effect on certain organisms such as *Strept. pyogenes* and if the delay between taking the swab and delivery to the laboratory is likely to be more than the limit stated then serum-coated swabs should be used. These prolong the survival time of bacteria on the swab.

The isolation rate for *Strept. pyogenes* is increased if a specimen of saliva, collected in a sterile universal container, is examined in addition to the throat swab.

Laboratory procedure
Bacteria which may be responsible for sore throat are *Strept. pyogenes*, Vincent's organisms and *C. diphtheriae*; thus the specimen should be inoculated on to the relevant diagnostic media.

1 *Strept. pyogenes.* Two plates of crystal violet blood agar (CVBA) are inoculated, a bacitracin disk is placed in the well-inoculum area of each, and one plate is incubated aerobically and the other under anaerobic conditions. The incorporation of a 1 in 500 000 concentration of crystal violet reduces the growth of commensal organisms; anaerobic conditions enhance the growth of *Strept. pyogenes* and if β-haemolytic streptococci grow on the plate but are inhibited in the vicinity of the bacitracin disk the strain very probably belongs to group A, i.e. *Strept. pyogenes*.

2 *C. diphtheriae.* A tube of Loeffler's inspissated serum medium and

a plate of tellurite medium are inoculated; the former gives very rapid growth from which films are made and stained by Gram's method and also to detect the presence of volutin granules, e.g. by Albert's method. Any growth showing Gram-positive bacilli which also possess volutin granules demands that the material from the Loeffler slope should be subinoculated to blood agar for further identification.

Growth of diphtheria bacilli is more slow on tellurite-containing media and films of colonies from such media do not always show volutin granules in the bacilli. Colonial morphology on tellurite media allows differentiation of the three biotypes of *C. diphtheriae* from each other and from commensal diphtheroid species.

All colonies suspected to be those of diphtheria bacilli must be examined for fermentative ability and then be used for tests demonstrating the production of diphtheria toxin.

3 *Vincent's organisms.* These organisms cannot be cultured for diagnostic purposes; hence the diagnosis of Vincent's infection depends on the microscopic demonstration of *large numbers* of *Borr. vincentii* and fusiform bacilli. Films are usually stained with dilute carbol fuchsin for 10 min.

In no other instance are films, made directly from the throat swab, of any diagnostic significance since the commensal flora of the throat and mouth are morphologically similar to and in some instances identical with the commonly encountered pathogens.

Crystal violet and tellurite are inhibitory substances and thus the swab or saliva should be inoculated on to Loeffler's media, CVBA and the tellurite medium in that order; then the film for Vincent's organisms is made.

SPUTUM

Although there are occasions when material from the lower respiratory tract can be obtained by bronchoscopy, most specimens comprise sputum coughed up from the bronchi. Sputum is therefore mixed with organisms in the throat and mouth before expectoration and many species may be present but in varying proportions.

It is important that the patient should be instructed that the specimen must be *coughed up* and that the material hawked from the post-nasal space or saliva are valueless.

In young children who cannot expectorate or in adults who are not producing sputum a laryngeal swab may be taken.

Delivery to the laboratory
Many of the species involved in chest infections have poor powers of survival outside the body, so that specimens must be processed in the laboratory within a few hours of being collected.

Laboratory procedure
Homogenization of the specimen must precede cultivation since by sampling different parts of the raw specimen different organisms are found; thus cultures made from homogenized sputum are much more representative of the total bacterial flora.

Homogenization can be effected either by adding sterile glass beads and vigorously shaking the specimen for 15–30 mins, or by the more efficient but more time-consuming pancreatin digestion technique. To the specimen is added an equal volume of 1% buffered pancreatin and the mixture is thoroughly shaken, then placed in a 37°C water bath for 1 hr during which time the mixture is thoroughly shaken every 15 min.

Thereafter a film is prepared and stained by Gram's method and two plates of blood agar medium are inoculated; one plate is incubated aerobically and the other in an atmosphere with a 5% concentration of CO_2. This latter plate assists the growth of *H. influenzae* and pneumococci; on both plates an 'Optochin' disk can be placed in the well inoculum area to give rapid differentiation of pneumococci from *Strept. viridans* and if a penicillin disk is also placed in the well inoculum it will inhibit many organisms in its immediate vicinity and give a selective zone in which any *H. influenzae* can grow, often in pure culture.

In cases of suspected pulmonary tuberculosis, at least six specimens of sputum should be examined. These are concentrated and the concentrate used to make films for staining by Ziehl-Neelsen's method and also to inoculate slopes of Lowenstein-Jensen's medium and guinea-pigs. In Britain nowadays many cases of pulmonary tuberculosis are detected at a much earlier stage in the illness and the tubercle bacilli are often much scantier than in established or chronic tuberculosis. Cultures should therefore be incubated for at least eight weeks before they are judged to be negative.

FAECES

Specimens of faeces are preferable to rectal swabs in the bacteriological investigation of cases of intestinal infection. A disadvantage of rectal swabs is that they are frequently not taken correctly and are only anal swabs; *it is essential* that the swab should pass into the rectum. Certain pathogenic species, including *Sh. sonnei* which is the commonest intestinal pathogen in Britain, do not survive for very long on plain cotton-wool swabs and therefore rectal swabs should be serum-coated; the use of rectal swabs denies *macroscopic* examination of the faeces and because of the small inoculum available for plating out etc, *microscopic* examination for the ova of protozoal parasites can be rarely undertaken.

Delivery to the laboratory
Specimens of faeces should be examined within a few hours of being collected and if the delay between collection and processing in the laboratory is likely to exceed 18–24 hr then the specimen should be thoroughly mixed with an equal volume of buffered glycerol-saline. Rectal swabs should be processed immediately they have been taken, hence their use should be restricted to the investigation of institutional outbreaks of intestinal infection when the swabs can be delivered to the laboratory within a very short time and before they have dried.

Laboratory procedure
Specimens of faeces are examined naked-eye for the presence of blood (fresh or altered), mucus and for any worms which may be present.
    Before any further examination is undertaken, any specimen which is solid or formed must be mixed with a quantity of sterile physiological saline sufficient to give a thick emulsion.

Microscopic examination
Gram-stained films of faeces are of no diagnostic value because of the morphological similarities between pathogens and the commensal coliforms in the gut. However, microscopic examination of wet film preparations will reveal the presence of pus cells and red blood cells as well as parasites and/or their ova.

Cultivation
Primarily the search is for shigellae and salmonellae which account for most cases of bacterial infection of the intestinal tract, thus plates of deoxycholate citrate agar (DCA) and MacConkey's medium are inoculated from the specimen. In addition to these selective media a sample of faeces should also be emulsified in tubes of two enrichment media, i.e. tetrathionate broth and selenite F broth; after these fluid enrichment media have been incubated for 12–18 hr at 37°C they are subinoculated to fresh DCA plates.

Any lactose non-fermenting (pale) colonies which appear on either DCA plate or on MacConkey's medium must be investigated for motility and fermentative reactions, and if such colonies give reactions typical for salmonellae or shigellae they must then be identified fully by serological methods.

Some laboratories also carry out routine procedures for the identification of enteropathogenic strains of *Esch. coli* whereas others do so only when requested; such strains grow poorly if at all on DCA but can be harvested from MacConkey's medium. Specimens suspected of containing enteropathogenic *Esch. coli* should also be plated out consecutively on two blood agar plates since some strains do not grow on MacConkey's medium.

There are no colonial or biochemical differences between commensal and enteropathogenic strains of *Esch. coli* so that the latter must be identified by serological methods. At least 10 colonies therefore must be tested by slide agglutination against a polyvalent serum prepared against the six enteropathogenic types and if any reaction is observed the colony is then checked with each of the individual specific antisera to allow type identification.

PUS AND WOUND DISCHARGES

Whenever possible, pus or excised tissue should be submitted for examination. The arrival of a single swab with a light smearing of dried pus accompanied by a request that the bacteriologist should search for pyogenic and anaerobic organisms causes much frustration and is unrealistic. Such swabs dry out very rapidly and many pathogenic species do not survive long, thus, *if swabs must be submitted*, they should be serum-coated and *at least three swabs from the one site* are required if the bacteriologist is to conduct a full investigation.

Dressings from discharging wounds or sinuses are acceptable specimens and should be transported in wide-mouthed, sterile, screw-capped containers e.g., honey pots.

Delivery to the laboratory
This should be as rapid as possible and if swabs or dressings are submitted they should be processed in the laboratory within 6–12 hr.

Laboratory procedure
1 *Macroscopic examination* should never be ignored; pus from streptococcal lesions is thin and serous in comparison with that from staphy-

lococcal infection, which frequently has a gelatinous appearance. In some instances pus resulting from infection with *Ps. pyocyanea* has a distinctive blue-green colour. In cases of actinomycosis sulphur granules may be noted; these may be semi-transparent or white if the lesion is early and the characteristic sulphur-yellow granules are seen in most chronic cases.

2   *Microscopic examination.* Films stained by Gram's method must always be examined; similarly a Ziehl-Neelsen-stained film should be prepared if the pus is from a suspected tuberculosis infection. If sulphur granules are seen then one should be crushed between two microscope slides, one slide then being stained by Gram's method and the other by Ziehl-Neelsen's method but substituting 1% H_2SO_4 for the 20% strength normally used.

3   *Cultivation.* All specimens must be cultured for pyogenic organisms by inoculating a blood agar plate and a plate of MacConkey's medium; thus the commonly encountered pyogenic organisms, i.e. *Staph. aureus* and *Strept. pyogenes* are readily isolated, as well as Gram-negative bacilli. A primary sensitivity plate should also be prepared.

In addition, either at the request of the clinician or because of the bacteriologist's suspicions (or intuition), a search may be made for anaerobic species. One must reiterate, however, that the recovery of a member of the genus *Clóstridium* from pathological material is not synonymous with clostridial infection and the diagnosis in all such cases rests solely with the clinician.

The attempted isolation of clostridium is a more sophisticated exercise, *and all media must be incubated under strictly anaerobic conditions.* A blood agar plate is inoculated and it is recommended that the agar content should be increased to 6% to discourage spreading of the clostridial colonies. A half-antitoxin plate may also be inoculated with the specimen. Several tubes of cooked-meat broth should be inoculated and then heated at 100°C for 5, 10 and 15 min before being incubated. Such heating destroys non-sporing pyogenic species so that they cannot contaminate either blood agar or half-antitoxin plates which are inoculated from the cooked-meat broths daily for one week. The latter are incubated throughout this period so that early subcultures will yield the rapidly growing clostridia and later subcultures cater for the more slowly growing members of the genus.

Solid media inoculated directly from the specimen or as subcultures from the cooked-meat broth must be incubated for at least 48 hr before the absence of growth allows a negative report to be issued.

CHAPTER 25
Antimicrobial sensitivity tests

In most people's minds the introduction of antimicrobial agents is equated with Domagk's discovery of the sulphonamides or even with the later discovery of the therapeutic value of penicillin which followed ten years after Fleming's original observations in the laboratory. However, antimicrobial agents have a much longer history even if one ignores the environmental uses of disinfectants and antiseptics.

Although the ancient Egyptians applied many medicaments topically the systemic administration of mercurial preparations in the attempted cure of syphilis was probably the first endeavour to eradicate deep-seated bacterial infection with an antagonistic agent.

Modern antimicrobial therapy was founded by Ehrlich, who studied the effects of dyestuffs on trypanosomes and showed that the latter could develop resistance to dyes which originally had been lethal. Ehrlich is best remembered, however, for his researches with salvarsan and its use in the treatment of syphilis. Ehrlich spoke of 'magic bullets' in the shape of antibodies or of drugs which could kill microorganisms in the patient's tissues but modern antimicrobial agents are more closely analogous to two-edged swords; no one could deny the benefits of chemotherapeutic or antibiotic drugs but at the same time the dangers associated with their abuse, and even their correct use, are not as widely appreciated.

The hazards of antimicrobial therapy can be classified into those affecting the individual patient and those affecting the community.

With regard to the treatment of a patient it is obvious that unless he is suffering from an infection caused by a microorganism that is sensitive to an antimicrobial agent there is no virtue in initiating such specific therapy. It has been reported that probably not more than 10% of the world's production of antibiotics is put to proper use. One can appreciate the pressures on the practitioner to prescribe anti-bacterial agents not only by pharmaceutical houses but by the patient or his parents or other relatives but such pressures cannot explain the use of these drugs for disorders like headache, toothache, sprained back etc, where they can have no merit whatsoever.

The need for a rational approach to the use of antibacterial drugs cannot be overstressed and the basis of this approach is that the clinician must make a diagnosis, at least provisionally, for each patient. There are certain infections which are caused only by one bacterial species, e.g. erysipelas, syphilis and yaws, and if there is no doubt of the *clinical diagnosis* in these and other such infections antibiotic therapy can be undertaken without laboratory guidance since the causal organisms are always sensitive to certain agents.

However, in many instances the clinical diagnosis may not be equated with a particular pathogen. For example, gastroenteritis may result from infection with bacteria, e.g. salmonellae and shigellae, or it may have a viral or protozoal aetiology and *in the majority of cases no acceptable pathogen can be indicted*. In this example the practitioner must certainly seek assistance from the microbiologist before instituting specific treatment.

A bacteriological diagnosis is essential in many other situations, e.g. sore throat syndrome, urinary tract infection, pneumonia and infections of burns and wounds; here, in any one patient, a variety of bacterial species may be involved and each may have differing sensitivities to antibiotics.

Thus the bacteriologist can assist the clinician by establishing which antimicrobial agent is most likely to help the patient's tissues to deal with the offending species.

Before outlining the laboratory procedures involved in sensitivity tests let us consider the *prophylactic* use of antimicrobial agents. There are a few clearcut indications for such a use and these include *long-term prophylactic administration* of penicillin to people known to have suffered from rheumatic fever. There is irrefutable evidence that such a régime protects against further episodes and thus minimizes any cardiac damage.

Short-term protection should also be given to any patient with con-genital or rheumatic heart disease when they undergo dental treatment so that any *Strept. viridans* which enter the blood stream are eliminated before they can settle on the damaged area of the heart where otherwise they may cause subacute bacterial endocarditis. Such protection must be given even if the dental treatment is of a conservative nature.

Other circumstances in which short-term protection or antibiotic 'cover' may be used include operations on the intestinal tract but here there is a division of opinion on the value offered; for *gastric* operations it is generally agreed that such cover is *harmful* since in several carefully controlled series, patients who did not receive any antibiotic had a significantly lower incidence of post-operative infections than patients given antibiotic cover. Such results are not surprising when we re- member that the stomach has a very scanty population of bacteria; on the other hand, the normal bacterial flora of the large intestine is im- mense so that *brief* administration of suitable antibiotics pre-operatively reduces the incidence of postoperative peritonitis *provided that* the anti- biotic cover is not used as an excuse for less exacting asepsis and surgical technique.

Apart from the above uses there are few indications for the prophy- lactic administration of antibiotics; the possible protection afforded to chronic bronchitics by 'winter month prophylaxis' with broad spectrum antibiotics has already been mentioned but the reputedly popular use of antibiotics to prevent secondary bacterial infection in patients suffering from virus infections is certainly unwise and may be danger- ous. In such patients it is better to withhold antibiotics and use them only in the few cases that become superinfected; possible exceptions to this rule are children suffering from hypogammaglobulinaemia or those who have serious congenital heart defects.

The indiscriminate use of antibiotics, therapeutically and prophy- lactically, is uneconomic and dangerous since patients are thus un- necessarily subjected to the risk of toxic side-effects or may develop hypersensitivity to an antibiotic which might in the future have been useful in treating some other infection. Similarly candidiasis and staphylococcal enterocolitis can arise if the normal flora is disturbed and these complications are severe and carry a high mortality rate.

Finally, the *community* may be subjected to unnecessary additional risks when antibiotic resistant strains evolve and can spread from the source; thus fresh cases of infection cannot receive the benefits of treat- ment with an antibiotic which otherwise would have assisted recovery. Perhaps the *community dangers* are best seen in regard to drug resistant strains of *Myco. tuberculosis*. The incidence of strains resistant to one or more of the therapeutically useful antituberculous drugs is high in those countries where laboratory control of therapy is non-existent or has been available only recently; thus not only in these countries but in others where the situation is much more satisfactory fresh cases of infection occur where the infecting strain can be tackled only with a diminishing therapeutic armamentarium and cases now occur where the drugs normally used—streptomycin, PAS and isoniazid—are of no value in treatment since the strain is resistant to all three.

Laboratory methods

It must be remembered that the *in vitro* testing of the activity of antibiotics against organisms isolated from pathological material is only a guide to their activity in the patient's tissues and that in the laboratory it is impossible to check the additional influences which the host defence mechanisms will have on the causal organism. This fact probably explains most instances where a satisfactory clinical response is obtained with an antibiotic which the bacteriologist has reported as being without effect, or having little influence, on the bacterial species involved.

Antibiotic sensitivity tests must be standardized with regard to various factors including *the size of inoculum* of the strain under test since by varying this it is possible with any one strain to demonstrate its extreme sensitivity to a given concentration of an antibiotic and by increasing the inoculum size to show that the same strain is resistant to the same concentration of that antibiotic. *The test medium* has a great influence on the results of testing antibiotic activity and its *composition, volume* and *pH* must be carefully specified otherwise great variation in results may be obtained, e.g. streptomycin has an activity at pH 8 which is more than 500 times its activity at a pH of 5.

The incubation time of the test must not exceed 18–24 hr since unstable antibiotics such as chlortetracycline will then appear less active.

Two methods of testing for antibiotic sensitivity are available:

Tube dilution method

Twofold dilutions of the antibiotic are prepared in a suitable fluid medium and each tube is then inoculated with a standard volume of bacterial suspension. Incubation is at 37°C for 18 hr and the series is then examined for turbidity in comparison with the growth in a control tube containing no antibiotic; *the bacteriostatic concentration* of the antibiotic is indicated by the tube with the highest dilution which shows no growth. *The bactericidal concentration* can be determined by subculturing from the tubes in which no growth is visible; aliquot volumes from these tubes are spread separately on agar plates so that residual antibiotic is diluted out and the plate is then incubated. The bactericidal concentration is that in the tube from which no growth is obtained on subculture.

The tube dilution method is too time-consuming for routine use and is reserved for special situations such as testing the sensitivity of slow-growing species such as *Myco. tuberculosis*.

Disk diffusion method

Here the strain to be tested is seeded evenly over the surface of nutrient agar in a Petri dish and when the surface of the medium is dry, filter paper disks containing the various antibiotics are placed on the medium into which the antibiotics diffuse and produce zones of inhibition of growth after incubation if the strain is sensitive.

Of course, the disks have to be of a standard diameter and thickness; 100 disks each 6·25 mm in diameter and punched from Whatman No. 1 filter paper will absorb 1 ml of fluid; hence if each antibiotic concentration is prepared, dispensed in 1 ml amounts and 100 disks are impregnated with such a volume then each disk will contain approximately 0·01 ml.

Similarly the depth of the medium is standardized by pouring a constant volume of medium into Petri dishes of constant diameter and obviously such plates must be poured on a horizontal surface to ensure uniformity of depth of the medium throughout each plate.

The bacterial inoculum may be from a broth culture or from a suspension of a colony from a culture plate and this is flooded over the surface of the medium; excess inoculum is removed with a Pasteur pipette and the surface is allowed to dry before disks are applied with sterile forceps. Since some antibiotics diffuse more slowly into the medium than do others a period of prediffusion before incubation gives more meaningful results; a period of 3–5 hr is recommended.

In practice there is no uniformity among laboratories in the amount of a particular antibiotic which should be incorporated in each disk but the amount must reflect a concentration which is attainable therapeutically in the patient's tissues.

Although disks are commonly employed as reservoirs in the diffusion method, other reservoirs from which the antibiotics can diffuse include holes punched out of the medium and porcelain or steel cylinders. These cylinders are placed on the surface and the relevant antibiotics are pipetted into them.

Since the size of the zones of inhibition differs with different antibiotics it is essential that standard graphs be prepared for each antibiotic. The graphs should relate, with regard to a standard organism, the zone sizes of inhibition obtained with varying concentrations of that antibiotic. Thus by measuring the diameter of the zone of inhibition of the antibiotic when it acts on a fresh isolate and then referring to a standard graph, the sensitivity of the isolate can be stated in units or μg/ml.

If the clinician wishes a more rapid guide to treatment then *primary* diffusion sensitivity tests can be performed. These differ from the sub-culture sensitivity tests described above only in that the inoculum comprises the pathological material which is spread over the medium as evenly as possible. Of course, in primary testing of sensitivity to anti-biotics we can have no control over the inoculum size and this causes difficulties in interpreting the results. However, the advantages, apart from speed, are that when more than one species is involved, e.g. in mixed infections of the urinary tract, the action of the antibiotics on two or more species is seen simultaneously, and also that around the disks selective zones often permit the growth of a resistant species in the zone of inhibition of a sensitive organism and thus allows separation of mixed cultures.

Bacteriologists make use of the varying sensitivities of different species to antimicrobial agents for diagnostic purposes; the use of 'Optochin' in differentiating pneumococci from *Strept. viridans* has been noted. Similarly strains of β-haemolytic streptococci belonging to group A are constantly sensitive to bacitracin, whereas strains belonging to other groups are rarely encountered as human pathogens and are resistant to this antibiotic. Thus if a bacitracin disk is placed in the well inoculum of a blood agar plate after inoculation with a throat swab or other material which may contain β-haemolytic streptococci, then in-hibition of characteristic colonies of these organisms allows a very rapid recognition of the human pathogenic members of group A with-out recourse to extraction of the group polysaccharide by chemical methods.

CHAPTER 26
Sterilization techniques

Apart from the use of antimicrobial agents in the treatment of bacterial infections there are many other occasions when we wish to kill microorganisms, e.g. the sterilization of syringes, surgical instruments and dressings, the provision of sterile media for the cultivation of other microorganisms and the terminal disinfection of a room (and its contents) which has been occupied by a case of smallpox or tuberculosis.

The method of sterilization employed depends primarily on the material being treated but regardless of the particular method used, sterilization is aimed at destroying all forms of microbial life.

Sterilization may be by *physical methods*, i.e. moist and dry heat, filtration or radiation, or alternatively by *chemical methods*.

PHYSICAL METHODS OF STERILIZATION

1 Dry heat
Here the death of microorganisms is caused by oxidation and charring.

(a) *Flaming to red heat* in a bunsen flame is a primitive but extremely efficient method of sterilizing inoculating loops in the laboratory, and *in an emergency* scalpels can be sterilized by dipping the blade in methylated spirits and then burning off the spirit; of course this process rapidly blunts the scalpel.

(b) *The hot air oven*, which is usually operated at 160°C for 1 hr, is invaluable for sterilizing glassware including assembled all-glass syringes; it is essential that the oven be loaded when it is at room temperature otherwise glassware may be cracked. Similarly after sterilization the temperature must be allowed to drop gradually before the oven is opened, not only because of the risk of breakage when glass is exposed to a sudden drop in temperature but also because contaminated cold air may pass through cotton wool stoppers.

Hot air ovens are basically two chambers, one within the other and the space between is thoroughly lagged with material, e.g. glass wool to reduce heat-loss; ovens are heated by gas or electricity and it is essential that the air inside should be circulated freely, e.g. by a fan, thus ensuring that the heated air is uniformly distributed; in the absence of some method of circulating the air the difference in temperature in different parts of the oven can be 20°C or 30°C—'hot air rises'.

2 Moist heat

Sterilization by moist heat is cheaper, quicker and more efficient than dry heat methods; moist heat sterilization kills microorganisms by co-agulative denaturation of their proteins. Moist heat can be applied under several conditions.

(a) *Boiling*. Whilst all vegetative cells are killed when subjected to boiling at 100°C for 10 min many sporing organisms can survive such treatment; the popular and almost ubiquitous domestic pressure cooker is much more efficient in sterilizing these articles which were previously 'sterilized' by boiling and should replace the latter method in general practice.

(b) *Pasteurization*. This method of heat-treating milk commemorates one of Pasteur's many discoveries. Pasteurization can be effected by either the *holder method* (63°C/30 min) or the *flash method* (72°C for 20 secs) and ensures the destruction of non-sporing bacteria, e.g. tubercle bacilli, members of the genus *Salmonella* and *Br. abortus* which, if present in milk, will not only survive but will multiply in such a rich medium.

(c) *Vaccine preparation*. Before most bacterial vaccines are issued for use they must be free from living bacteria; the temperature and time employed must be adequate to destroy bacteria but at the same time must be low enough to have a minimal destructive effect on the anti-genic material. Vaccines are usually treated at 60°C for 1 hr, and must be subjected to vigorous tests of sterility before being used.

(d) *Sterilization of culture media*. Many of the media used in the laboratory cannot be subjected to autoclaving since their constituents would be altered sufficiently to render the media valueless for their in-tended purpose. In such instances sterility is assured by the use of the Koch steamer; here the material is exposed to steam at atmospheric pressure for 30 min on 3 consecutive days. The first steaming kills off all vegetative forms of bacteria and since the medium is left at room temperature for 24 hr before the second steaming any bacterial spores present will germinate and the emergent cells will be destroyed by the second steaming; the third and final steaming is intended as a precautionary measure.

(e) *Autoclaving.* By employing saturated steam under increased pressure temperatures above 100°C can be attained and this method is the only one which ensures the total destruction of all microorganismal life including the most highly resistant spores.

As in other methods of sterilization the materials to be treated must be suitably covered to prevent re-contamination after they have been sterilized and the covering must be of a type which allows steam to penetrate to the wrapped materials and also to allow drying of the materials after sterilization. Details of the construction and operation of the several types of autoclave should be sought in specialized textbooks but some important rules are given below.

1   Autoclaves must be fitted with a thermometer and a steam pressure gauge since only by checking that both temperature *and* pressure are at the desired levels can one be certain that sterilizing conditions have been attained.

2   The articles to be sterilized must be loaded into the autoclave in a manner that ensures even and complete exposure to the steam.

3   Some method of checking sterility should be incorporated in each load being autoclaved; chemical methods are frequently used, e.g. Browne's sterilizer control tubes which show a colour change from red to green when exposed to various combinations of temperature and duration of exposure. Biological methods of checking the efficiency of the sterilization process may also be employed but are more time-consuming as they involve the attempted isolation of organisms, e.g. *Bacillus stearothermophilus* after its spores have been included in a pack being autoclaved.

3 Filtration

Several types of filter are available which allow the retention of bacteria when broth cultures or other fluids, e.g. water, flow through them. Thus we can harvest bacterial exotoxins separately from the organisms which produced them and similarly fluids such as serum which would be coagulated by heat sterilization methods can be rendered free from bacteria.

The earlier types of *earthenware filters*, e.g. Berkefeld, have been largely replaced by other kinds. The *Seitz filter* is made of asbestos, *sintered glass filters* are made of small ground glass particles fused together and several grades of porosity are available in all of these filters. However, *membrane filters* (made of cellulose acetate) have many advantages over other filters; the rate of filtration is much more rapid, their porosity is much more exact and uniform and they are much less absorptive, so that in the collection of exotoxins the potency of the filtrate is much greater than with other types of filter.

Furthermore, by placing the used membrane filter on a suitable culture medium bacteria retained on the surface can be grown and their colonies identified, e.g. large volumes of water can be processed through a membrane filter and the presence of any pathogenic bacteria be recognized.

Since, even with membrane filters, gravity filtration is slow it is normal practice to use positive or more usually negative pressure to assist filtration.

4 Radiation

Many bacteria are killed fairly rapidly when they are exposed to direct sunlight and this lethal action is due essentially to ultraviolet radiation; such radiation is used artificially to reduce the population of bacteria in the air under certain circumstances, e.g. in ampouling chambers in the pharmaceutical industries. *Gamma radiation.* Gamma rays from a Cobalt 60 source are being used increasingly for the sterilization of many materials, e.g. plastic disposable syringes. In spite of the cost of installing such a plant the efficiency of the method has encouraged industry to make increasing use of gamma radiation. A particular advantage is that there is little appreciable rise in the temperature of materials being sterilized although the time required for sterilization is 36–48 hr. As a check on the irradiation process a polyvinyl chloride envelope containing an azo dye is included and chlorine is liberated by the action of the gamma rays and this results in a colour change from yellow to red.

CHEMICAL METHODS OF STERILIZATION

Many chemicals are used to destroy bacteria and their spores and it is customary to classify these into *disinfectants* and *antiseptics*. Disinfectants are 'stronger' and are used only on inanimate material, whereas antiseptics are less irritant and can be applied to human tissues since their cytotoxic activity is relatively greater on microorganisms than against the protoplasm of skin and mucous membranes.

Several methods of assessing the antibacterial activity of disinfectants have been established but all of them are unrealistic to a greater or lesser extent as they cannot reproduce the natural circumstances in which disinfectants and antiseptics are used. For example, such tests do not take into account the number of organisms to be killed, nor do they adequately allow for the deviation of the disinfectant by organic material other than bacteria. Similarly the much greater resistance of bacterial spores as compared with vegetative cells is not tested.

In the following paragraphs there is presented a résumé of the use of various chemical methods of killing bacteria.

1 Phenols and cresols

'Lysol' (Liquor cresolis saponatus) is widely used domestically and in hospitals as a disinfectant; it is more surface-active than carbolic acid by virtue of its possessing alkyl groups larger than C_6H_5. Phenol and its homologues and analogues are relatively unaffected by the presence of organic matter such as pus or faeces; in 0·5% concentration phenol is used as a preservative for serum and vaccines.

2 Dye-stuffs

Prior to the discovery of antibiotics certain dyes, e.g. gentian violet, were used in the treatment of skin infections due to Gram-positive cocci; they are relatively non-toxic to human tissues but are easily in-activated by non-bacterial proteins.

Dyes are incorporated in certain culture media which are thus made relatively selective, e.g. crystal violet is added to blood agar and allows β-haemolytic streptococci to grow and at the same time discourages the growth of staphylococci; similarly malachite green, present in Lowen-stein-Jensen's medium has no action against tubercle bacilli but deters the growth of many rapidly growing contaminants.

3 Halogens

Following on filtration, water supplies for domestic use, e.g. for drinking or in swimming pools, are disinfected with chlorine which is added in the proportion 1–2 parts/10^6; thus hypochlorous acid is formed and is rapidly bactericidal.

Iodine as a 2% solution in 70% alcohol is popular as a disinfecting agent for skin before surgical operations.

4 Alcohols

Absolute ethyl alcohol has a very weak disinfectant action but its activity improves dramatically when diluted with water and a 70% concentration of ethyl alcohol is optimal as a disinfecting agent; such a concentration is widely employed to clean skin before an injection is given.

5 Soaps and synthetic detergents

Whilst these have reasonable bactericidal properties their primary action is the removal of microorganisms from skin and other surfaces. Cationic detergents have a wider antibacterial action than soaps and anionic detergents and the latter are much more active against Gram-positive cocci and have little activity against Gram-negative species. It must be remembered that the cationic detergents, e.g. cetrimide, are in-activated by soaps and anionic detergents so that they must not be used in combination.

There are many other classes of chemical agents which have a disinfectant or antiseptic action but two agents require particular mention.

Formaldehyde

This extremely efficient antimicrobial agent is also sporicidal. It is used in the laboratory at a concentration of 0·5–1·0% to kill bacteria, e.g. in the preparation of bacterial suspensions for use in agglutination tests such as the Widal reaction.

It deserves wider use in terminal disinfection of premises occupied by cases of tuberculosis, smallpox, anthrax, etc. since not only is it cheap but it does not harm fabrics, e.g. cloth, leather, wool, etc. Formaldehyde is, however, an irritant to human tissues and it must be used carefully; since the gas is water soluble it is frequently used as a 40% solution in water ('Formalin').

Very recently the combination of sub-atmospheric steam and formaldehyde has been introduced for the sterilization of many heat-sensitive items; treatment in a high vacuum autoclave at a sub-atmospheric pressure yields steam at 70–80°C and, along with 5 ml of Formalin per cubic foot, will achieve sterilization of items thus exposed in 2 hr.

Ethylene oxide

Sterilization of materials which are heat sensitive has always presented a problem and the relatively recent introduction of ethylene oxide has solved this problem. It is extremely active against all microbial life including bacterial spores. Because it forms an explosive mixture in air special techniques must be used. These usually involve the use of special chambers in which a high vacuum can be drawn before the ethylene oxide is introduced at a concentration of 10% in CO_2 and at a pressure of 5–25 lb/in^2 above atmospheric pressure. Perhaps the only disadvantage in using ethylene oxide is the long exposure—several hours

—which is required for sterilization but it is undoubtedly the method of choice for many materials, e.g. plastics, endoscopes and heart–lung machines. Ethylene oxide is toxic to human tissues, and since the gas may be absorbed into material thus sterilized, it is essential that the sterile material is stored for five or more days after treatment to allow any absorbed gas to escape.

It must be stressed that in using any method of sterilization *the materials to be treated must be thoroughly cleaned* BEFORE *being sterilized*; if this preliminary treatment is not given then even vegetative bacterial cells may survive the sterilizing process since they can be protected by a layer of dried pus or other filth.

VIROLOGY

CHAPTER 27
Introduction

In 1884, at a time when bacteria were being discovered and causally associated with infection in man and animals, Pasteur suspected that even smaller agents, or viruses as we now call them, were the cause of rabies since he was unable to detect bacteria in infective material from rabid dogs. Then in 1892 Ivanowsky determined that the agent causing mosaic disease in tobacco plants was ultramicroscopic and could pass through bacteria-stopping filters; thus the flood gates opened and the presence of similar filter-passing, ultramicroscopic organisms, was demonstrated in many diseases including foot and mouth disease (1898), yellow fever (1901) and even in association with tumour production in fowls in 1911.

Not only do viruses affect animals, plants and insects and cause economic havoc in addition to causing human infections, but bacteria can also be infected by ultramicroscopic, filter-passing particles and these agents, described independently by Twort (1915) and d'Herelle (1917), are termed bacteriophages.

In the last 30–40 years many more features of viruses have been established and in contrast to bacteria, the vast majority of viruses are not only ultramicroscopic in terms of the light microscope and able to pass through bacteria-stopping filters, but possess the following distinguishing characteristics:

1 They possess *only* DNA *or* RNA—not both.
2 They do not possess ribosomes or mitochondria.
3 They do not have a rigid cell wall.
4 They do not undergo binary fission.
5 They cannot synthesize the macromolecules they require.
6 They reproduce only within host cells and thus are the ultimate parasites.

7   They are insensitive to antibiotics.

8   They are sensitive to interferon.

In their epidemiological behaviour they are very similar to other microorganisms, in that they share methods of spread from host to host and any one virus can cause infection of varying severity and also be carried without ill effect on the host—a feature of viruses usually termed *latency*. Similarly, virus infections may be zoonotic, e.g. rabies.

A few viruses are *oncogenic*, i.e. produce tumours, and several undoubted examples in animals have been added to the original discovery by Rous in 1911 that fowl sarcoma could be transmitted by cell-free filtrates of the tumour. In man only one proven example exists at present, i.e. the causal role of papovavirus in infectious warts; however, the probable association of Burkitt's lymphoma with a virus and a possible link between cervical carcinoma and a herpesvirus have generated even greater interest in the prospect of a viral aetiology in human neoplasms.

CLASSIFICATION

As yet there is no satisfactory scheme of classifying viruses although there have been several attempts to do so, on a scientific taxonomic basis. Because a virus possesses only DNA *or* RNA a simple subdivision can be made as shown in the Table and within these two categories, groups of viruses are recognized on other criteria, e.g. size, design, susceptibility to physical/chemical agents.

It is worth recalling at this point the effects of physical and chemical agents on viruses; most viruses are inactivated at 56°C for 30 min although some, e.g. papovaviruses, can resist such exposure. By contrast, viruses are stable at low temperatures, e.g. −70°C, although a few are partially inactivated by lyophilization. UV irradiation inactivates viruses but many can survive drying, e.g. smallpox virus, whilst others are rapidly killed. As noted in the Table, some viruses, i.e. those containing lipid, are sensitive to ether.

Such factors have a practical influence regarding the collection and transport of specimens since many viruses may survive only a few hours outside the body so that specimens must reach the laboratory with the minimum delay otherwise the specimens must be frozen.

Whilst the resistance of true viruses to sulphonamides and antibiotics is useful in allowing the virologist to 'purify' virus-containing material, e.g. sputum, from bacterial contaminants, there are virucidal agents available for sanitizing virus infected materials and of these, oxidizing

SOME MEDICALLY IMPORTANT VIRUSES

	Features	*Diseases*
DNA VIRUSES		
1. Poxviruses	Brick shaped with complex symmetry	Smallpox
		Cowpox
	Sensitive to ether	Vaccinia
	Resists drying	Molluscum contagiosum
2. Adenoviruses	Naked icosahedron	Latent infections
	Resistant to ether	Mild respiratory diseases
		Pharyngo-conjunctival fever
3. Herpesviruses	Enveloped icosahedron	Latent infection
	Sensitive to ether	Chickenpox, shingles, herpes simplex
		Stomatitis
		? Glandular fever
		? Burkitt's tumour
4. Papovaviruses	Icosahedron	Infective warts
	Resistant to ether	
	Heat resistant	
RNA VIRUSES		
1. Orthomyxoviruses	Enveloped	Influenza
	Spherical or filamentous	Pneumonia,–? bronchitis
	Sensitive to ether	
2. Paramyxoviruses	Enveloped and pleomorphic	Acute respiratory infection
	Larger than orthomyxoviruses	Mumps, measles
	Sensitive to ether	
3. Rhabdoviruses	Enveloped, bullet-shaped helical	Rabies
	Sensitive to ether	
4. Arboviruses	Enveloped	Yellow fever
	Sensitive to ether	Dengue fever
	Arthropod borne	Encephalitis
5. Picorna viruses	Naked icosahedron	Poliomyelitis
	Resistant to ether	Bornholm disease
		Carditis
		Common cold

agents, e.g. hydrogen peroxide and potassium permanganate, are the most useful.

In the field, formaldehyde vapour in proper concentrations is the agent for disinfection of premises which have been used in the disinfection of apparatus used in renal dialysis units.

STRUCTURE OF VIRUSES

Virion is the term used to describe a complete infectious virus particle and it comprises strands of DNA *or* RNA sheathed with a protein coat, i.e. the *capsid* which is structured from sub-units termed *capsomeres*. The capsid offers protection to the contained nucleic acid or genome from damage or destruction by external agencies, e.g. host defence mechanisms. Virions may also have an ultimate exterior cover of lipoprotein, the *envelope*, which is largely derived from the outer membrane of the host cell; in some instances, e.g. herpesvirus, the envelope is acquired from the altered nuclear membrane of the host cell.

Morphologically there are three kinds of virus structure as revealed by electronmicroscopy; *helical* viruses, e.g. influenza and rabies viruses, in which the virus particle is elongate or cylindrical and wound in the form of a helix or spiral. *Isometric* viruses, e.g. herpesviruses, are those where the capsid takes the form of an icosahedron and the third type is the *complex* virus particle, e.g. pox virus, which does not conform to helical or isometric symmetry.

Some viruses, notably the orthomyxoviruses, have projecting prickles or spikes which attach to specific receptors when the virus is mixed with red blood cells and haemagglutination is observed; these haemagglutinin spikes are triangular in cross section in contrast to mushroom-shaped protein projections possessing the enzyme neuraminidase.

LABORATORY DIAGNOSIS

As in bacterial infections the microbiologist aims at accuracy and speed in identifying viral agents in cases of infection; because of our inability to treat specifically most viral infections laboratory diagnosis may not seem relevant but epidemiological prospects, particularly the use of control measures dictates the need for identification. Fortunately, many virus infections give classical pictures, e.g. measles, and material from such infections is rarely submitted for laboratory investigation but contrarily the need to distinguish cases of chickenpox from atypical smallpox cases has stimulated the introduction of very rapid and reliable methods of identifying the causal agents.

Microscopic examination

The use of the *electron microscope* particularly in the differentiation of smallpox and chickenpox viruses obtained from skin lesions is invaluable; it must be noted, however, that large numbers of virions must be present in the specimen and that failure to demonstrate virus particles does *not* exclude a diagnosis of viral infection.

Similarly the demonstration of virus particles in a specimen may be undertaken by *fluorescent antibody tests*, usually by the indirect technique; here again a rapid diagnosis can be made and with fewer virions present per ml of specimen. However, as with most fluorescent antibody methods, non-specific reactions may cause difficulties and control preparations must be viewed in parallel to eliminate the risk of false positive results.

Finally at the microscopic level a few viruses are sufficiently large to be seen in stained smears viewed under the oil-immersion objective of the compound light microscope.

Isolation of viruses

Since viruses will grow only inside living host cells special techniques have been evolved to cater for them, and at present the most widely used method for virus isolation is that of *cell culture*.

Animal and human tissue cells can be grown and maintained *in vitro* provided that their nutritional requirements are met; their maintenance *in vitro* is enhanced by incorporating certain antibiotics, e.g. penicillin and streptomycin, to eliminate bacterial contamination. Of the tissue cells used in cell culture, monkey kidney, human amnion and chick embryo are the most common; cells are dispersed by trypsin and then distributed into test tubes or other suitable vessels containing nutrient medium. The cells settle on the glass surface and during incubation grow to form a continuous monolayer; such *primary* cell cultures can then be detached from the glass by trypsin and seeded into fresh medium where they continue to divide and can be subcultured. These *secondary* cell cultures may be maintained under carefully controlled conditions for 50 or more subcultures before they die. On occasion such cell cultures spontaneously undergo transformation to become an *established cell line* which grows more rapidly than the parent cell and cells from an established line can be subcultured indefinitely.

DETECTION OF VIRUSES IN TISSUE CULTURES

Cytopathic effect (CPE)
Many viruses alter the appearance of the infected cells in tissue culture
and such changes can be noted by examining the monolayer intermittently with the low-power objective in a light microscope. The CPE
varies with different viruses and the speed with which CPE may be
noted also varies from a few hours to several weeks. Regardless of the
type of CPE produced it spreads throughout all of the cells in the
monolayer which is eventually destroyed.

Some viruses do not produce a CPE and their presence in tissue
culture cells is then detected indirectly.

Haemagglutination
Viruses not producing a CPE but possessing a haemagglutinin can be
spotted by testing the cell culture fluid for ability to agglutinate a suspension of suitable red blood cells.

Haemadsorption
Haemagglutinating viruses which are formed at the host cell cytoplasmic
membrane can be detected by adding erythrocytes to infected tissue
cultures where they adhere to infected cells.

Interference
Host cells infected with non CPE-producing viruses cannot be infected
when challenged with a second virus known to give a CPE. Thus the
absence of CPE after the second inoculation infers the existence of an
earlier viral inoculum.

Fluorescence
As in the microscopic examination of patients' specimens, infected
tissue culture cells not showing a CPE can be examined by immunofluorescence using a specific antiserum for the infecting virus.

Other systems can be used in the attempted isolation of viruses from
specimens.

Animal inoculation
This was the technique originally used but it suffered disadvantages;
adult animals may have acquired natural immunity to viruses and

animals also carry viruses and these may either prevent replication of the experimentally inoculated virus or alternatively the latter virus may stimulate clinical infection by the latent virus. Only in the case of arboviruses and coxsackie A viruses are animals used in attempted isolation; for both viruses suckling mice are used since these will not have acquired immunity to either of the groups of viruses.

Chick embryo
Although the introduction in the early 1930s of embryonated hens' eggs for virus isolation was a distinct advance since fertile eggs do not possess antibody, they may carry fowl leukosis viruses. However, the chick embryo is not susceptible to as many viruses as tissue culture cells. The main routes of inoculation are into the amniotic or allantoic cavity and on to the chorioallantoic membrane.

Detection of viruses in the chick embryo is either direct by noting the formation of lesions (pocks) on the inoculated chorioallantoic membrane or indirectly by detecting haemagglutination in fluid withdrawn from the amniotic or allantoic cavities.

Inoculation of the chorioallantoic membrane is the only method of distinguishing variola and vaccinia viruses from each other and from chickenpox virus.

SEROLOGY

The demonstration of the acquisition of viral antibody during a patient's illness may be of diagnostic significance either alone or complementing microscopic detection of viruses in specimens and/or their isolation by one or other of the methods outlined above. It is preferable to demonstrate a significant rise in antibody titre by testing a serum specimen obtained during the acute phase of illness along with a second specimen of serum taken 10–14 days after the first specimen; a fourfold or greater rise in a doubling dilution system is regarded as significant. Not infrequently a viral aetiology for an illness is not contemplated until the patient is convalescing and a retrospective diagnosis may be requested by the clinician on the basis of a single, convalescent specimen of serum and if the titre of antibody for a particular virus is significantly high many clinicians happily accept such a finding to clinch their clinical diagnosis.

Of the serological techniques used for detecting antibody *complement fixation* is most commonly employed by diagnostic virologists and the basis of the test is identical with that used in bacteriological diagnosis.

Neutralization tests are also used but are more expensive and time-consuming than other methods. Here serial dilutions of the patient's serum are mixed with a standard infective dose of the particular virus and neutralization of the infective dose is assayed by challenging tissue cultures, chick embryos or animals and the highest dilution of serum that inhibits infectivity is noted as the neutralizing titre of antibody.

Haemagglutination inhibition tests can be used to assay antibody against viruses that produce a haemagglutinin by noting the highest dilution of the patient's serum that inhibits haemagglutination by a stock haemagglutinating virus.

As in serological tests with bacterial antigens all tests for viral antibodies must incorporate suitable controls to eliminate false reactions.

CHAPTER 28
Poxviruses

SMALLPOX

Smallpox is the most significant infection caused by the pox group of viruses and although endemic infection no longer occurs in Britain and many other countries there is a constant danger of epidemics arising from importation of cases from these countries, e.g. in Asia, where the disease still thrives. This risk is heightened by air travel which allows cases in the incubation period (on average 12 days) to become resident in a non-endemic area before the infection declares itself.

Smallpox does occur in vaccinated individuals and usually in a modified form which may be missed or mistaken for chickenpox (varicella); such modified cases have been the source of epidemics in Britain and constitute one example of why we must increasingly and continuously 'think globally', not only in the epidemiological sense but in regard to individual patients whether immigrant or those who, on business or vacation, have been resident abroad.

A case can act as a source of infection to others from the time that the skin rash appears and this occurs simultaneously with pathologically identical lesions in the upper respiratory tract; infection is acquired by inhalation of respiratory secretions or from bedding or other fomites. It must be noted that the variola virus is tough and can survive outside the host for weeks or months provided it is protected, e.g. as in the crusts shed from the patient's skin lesion; thus smallpox is one of the few infections in which thorough current and terminal disinfection must be undertaken.

The viruses
The variola virus of classical smallpox (variola major) is morphologically identical with that causing alastrim (variola minor) and with the

179

vaccinia virus used for vaccination against smallpox and these all appear as large brick-shaped virions under the electron microscope. These complex particles are sufficiently large (200–300nm) to be visible in stained preparations viewed by the compound light microscope.

Other features common to these viruses and to the cowpox and other animal poxviruses are sensitivity to ether, growth in tissue culture (e.g. monkey kidney) with a 'ballooning' CPE effect in the cells and also the ability to haemagglutinate fowl RBCs.

However, although all poxviruses produce pocks on the chorio-allantoic membrane of chick embryos the viruses produce different and characteristic lesions.

Laboratory diagnosis

Microscopy
Scrapings from the early maculo-pupular-lesions, from the base of vesicles or crusts formed later in the illness can all be used and ideally the material should be examined by *electron microscopy* to visualize the virus particles; although the viruses of smallpox, vaccinia and cowpox are identical in appearance they will not be confused with the ico-sahedron virions of chickenpox or herpes simplex. A result can be obtained within 15 min of the specimen reaching the laboratory.

Material taken from lesions up to the clear vesicle stage of the disease can also be smeared on to slides and stained (e.g. with Gutstein's stain) and a search made for elementary bodies by *light microscopy*; because of the amount of pus and other debris present in lesions at and beyond the pustular stage of illness this method cannot then be employed.

Serology
Complement fixation and gel-diffusion tests, using material from the lesions as the antigen, can also detect the common viral antigen present in variola, vaccinia and other poxviruses and will differentiate between the pox group antigen and those of varicella and herpes simplex.

Cultivation
The lesions produced on the inoculated chorioallantoic membrane of the chick embryo allow differentiation of the smallpox viruses from those of vaccinia and varicella.

The *smallpox viruses* produce small white discrete pocks 2 mm in diameter 48–72 hr after inoculation; ability to grow at 38·5°C differentiates the virus of classical smallpox from that causing alastrim.

Vaccinia virus produces large, diffuse grey pocks with necrotic centres when grown on the chorioallantoic membrane and varicella virus does not produce lesions.

Control of smallpox

Vaccination by the multiple pressure method remains the sheet anchor of preventive measures in smallpox. Isolation of cases with current and terminal disinfection of premises and their contents is vital in prevention of spread and it is essential that the clinician, the Medical Officer of Health and the microbiologist collaborate fully in tracing and checking on contacts of the case and keeping them under surveillance.

Inner ring contacts are those who have been close to the patient and should be immediately vaccinated or re-vaccinated and also offered human gamma globulin obtained from recently vaccinated individuals. More recently the proven value of methisazone in protecting contacts demands that it should be given to close contacts. Since these measures may modify smallpox should it occur in an inner ring contact they must be under close clinical surveillance and indeed the isolation of close contacts during the last 3–4 days of the possible incubation period of the disease is advocated; thus should such contacts develop smallpox, in spite of preventive measures, they will not then act as fresh sources of infection.

Outer ring contacts who have not been close to the case but simply have been in contact with inner ring contacts or have been in the same general environment as the primary case should be offered vaccination but their surveillance need not otherwise be so strict.

CHAPTER 29
Adenoviruses

The first isolation of these viruses was from adenoid tissue—hence their group name; so far 33 serotypes have been recognized and these have been incriminated as the cause of pharyngitis and conjunctivitis and they also exist without obvious pathological changes in lymphoid tissue throughout the body.

Certain serotypes have been shown to be oncogenic in experimental animals but there is no evidence that they are associated with tumours in man.

Pharyngo-conjunctival fever is the usual epidemic expression of adenoviruses—the illness lasts for 5–7 days and is characterized by fever, pharyngitis and conjunctivitis; epidemics are not infrequently seen in schools, residential nurseries, holiday camps and military establishments and occur most commonly in summer and types 3, 4, 7 and 14 are most often incriminated.

Acute respiratory disease, caused mainly by the same serotypes, is a coryzal illness of epidemic occurrence usually in semi-closed communities.

Epidemic kerato-conjunctivitis is caused only by serotype 8 and is a serious infection often spread by contaminated ophthalmic instruments and therapeutic solutions. The colloquial term 'ship-yard eye' emphasizes the importance of industrial eye injuries, requiring treatment at eye clinics, in precipitating this adenovirus infection which can then be spread to the patient's family via communal fomites in the home, e.g. hand towels.

Endemic infection with adenoviruses occurs in the open community and accounts for about 10% of minor respiratory tract infections. Outside the respiratory tract their tropism for lymphoid tissue is emphasized by the isolation of adenoviruses from enlarged intestinal

glands excised during appendicectomy in cases of mesenteric lympha-
denitis in children; similarly they may play an indirect role in intus-
susception which may result from increased peristalsis on enlarged
intestinal glands.

More than half of the serotypes of adenovirus seem to inhabit the
intestinal tract but their significance in the gut has still to be elucidated.

The viruses

These are morphologically identical, icosahedral particles (60–70nm in
diameter); 12 fibres with terminal knobs project from the vertices of
the icosahedron. Resistant to ether and agglutinate a variety of RBCs;
can be grouped according to ability to agglutinate RBCs of rat and/or
rhesus monkey, e.g. type 8 strains agglutinate both types of RBC,
types 3, 7 and 14 agglutinate only rhesus monkey RBCs whereas
type 4 strains do not affect rhesus RBCs but partially agglutinate rat
erythrocytes.

Grow slowly in a variety of tissue cultures and infected cells become
rounded, swell to about twice their size and then cluster into bunches
like grapes.

Laboratory diagnosis

Specimens, e.g. mouth washings, are inoculated on to tissue culture,
preferably of human amnion and CPE observed after 1–4 days. Confirmation of the virus as an adenovirus is sought by complement fixation tests with standard antisera; the *group* to which the isolate belongs
can then be determined by testing its haemagglutinating activities with
rat and rhesus monkey erythrocytes. Finally the *serotype* can be recognized by neutralization tests with specific antiserum.

Complement fixation tests with paired sera, using the common group
antigen, and the detection of a significant rise in titre affords serological
evidence of adenovirus infection.

Control

The endemic nature of many adenovirus infections combined with the
mildness of the infection has not encouraged the development of
vaccines except on an experimental basis. Obviously there is a need for
control of shipyard eye (type 8 virus) by ensuring sterility of instruments, medicaments, etc., in ophthalmic clinics.

CHAPTER 30
Herpesviruses

HERPES SIMPLEX INFECTION, CHICKENPOX, SHINGLES

HERPES SIMPLEX INFECTIONS

Primary infection with *Herpesvirus hominis* is symptomless in most instances and occurs between 1–3 yrs of age; when the primary infection declares itself clinically it is almost invariably as a gingivo-stomatitis with vesicles on the buccal mucosa; the illness is distressing to the infant who is febrile and pathetic in its unwillingness to feed or be free from pain but healing occurs in 7–14 days. The conjunctivae or the cornea or the genitalia may also be the site of primary infection in infants. More rare and often severe primary infections include herpetic whitlow, most often seen in nurses and sometimes in epidemic form; generalized infection may occur in new-born children of mothers who did not possess serum antibodies and in such instances the neonate is infected from others involved in its care.

Eczema herpeticum, i.e. superinfection of eczematous lesions may also be caused by *Herpesvirus hominis* and may be difficult to distinguish from eczema vaccinatum due to the vaccinia virus; both instances of superinfection of eczema are entitled Kaposi's varicelliform eruption. Finally and fortunately rarely, the herpesviruses may show their neurotropic nature and primary infection may present as meningo-encephalitis or acute necrotizing encephalitis which carry a very poor prognosis.

Recurrent infection with the herpes virus is commonly seen as herpes labialis or cold sore recurring at the same site and usually at muco-cutaneous junctions on the lips or at the nostrils but any mucous

184

membrane and any part of the skin may be involved. Between recurrences the virus is latent in host cells in spite of the individual's high level of serum antibody and reactivation is often associated with the individual suffering some respiratory infection.

The virus
Icosahedral in shape, medium sized (120nm), sensitive to ether and as well as infecting a variety of animals grows readily in many types of tissue culture and on the chorioallantoic membrane of embryonated hens eggs. Growth on the latter allows two types of herpes virus to be identified; type 1 virus produces white pocks less than 0·75 mm, whereas type 2 virus strains give pocks of at least 1 mm in diameter. The two virus types can also be separated by neutralization tests and they differ in other features, e.g. thermolability; there is also a fascinating difference in their association with human lesions since type 1 strains are isolated essentially from the mouth, eye and CNS and in skin lesions above the waist, whereas type 2 strains are recovered mainly from genital lesions and skin vesicles occurring from the waist downwards!

Laboratory diagnosis
Vesicle fluid or scrapings from the base of lesions are used.

Microscopy
Although typical virions can be seen electron microscopically this method does not differentiate herpesviruses from that of chickenpox. Immunofluorescent staining with herpes-specific antibody may be used.

Cultivation
Tissue culture cells of several types produce a typical ballooning and rounding within 24–48 hours of inoculation with material containing herpesvirus. Inoculation of the chorioallantoic membranes of chick embryos yields white pocks within 2–3 days and the pock size after further incubation allows the virus type to be recognized and the type identification can be confirmed by neutralization tests with standard antisera.

Serology
The detection of a rising titre of complement fixing antibodies is useful in the diagnosis of *primary* infections but the continuing presence of antibodies thereafter renders such a method valueless in the diagnosis of recurring infections.

Treatment
Idoxuridine applied topically is successful in the treatment of herpetic eye infection, reducing the severity of the lesion and the duration of the illness; it has also been used systemically in attempted treatment of herpes encephalitis, but reports of its value here are conflicting.

Prevention
The symptomless nature of the majority of cases of primary infection and the almost universal nature of the infection denies any prospect of prophylactic measures being successful. Obviously eczematous children should be protected from contact with people suffering cold sores or other children suffering gingivostomatitis.

CHICKENPOX/SHINGLES
(Varicella/Zoster)

These two diseases are *caused by the same virus*, the Varicella-Zoster (V-Z) virus; chickenpox is the primary infection and recurrent infection declares itself as shingles.

Chickenpox is one of the more infectious but also one of the mildest infections in childhood, and its significance lies mainly in its occasional similarity to smallpox and the fact that when chickenpox does occur in adults it is usually more severe than in childhood where the infection is usually nothing more than a tiresome and irritating episode to patient and parent alike.

Shingles on the other hand is mainly a disease of adults, and unlike the widespread centripetally distributed rash of chickenpox the vesicles in shingles are restricted in distribution to the area of one or two sensory nerves—commonly on the thorax and often unilaterally and it also involves the cranial nerves. Shingles is due to reactivation of latent virus following chickenpox.

The virus
The V-Z virus is larger (150–200nm) than the herpes simplex virus and is identical with the latter electron microscopically. Does not grow in the chick embryo but gives focal lesions with multinucleated giant cells when grown on human tissue culture cells, e.g. embryo lung cultures. Although V-Z virus is cell-free in vesicle fluid from cases of chickenpox and shingles it remains cell associated in tissue culture.

Laboratory diagnosis

The only occasion when this is indicated is where there is need for rapid differentiation between chickenpox and smallpox (see Chapter 28).

Prevention

Chickenpox is clinically a mild infection but highly contagious and may be spread by droplet infection from saliva or from fomites contaminated from vesicular lesions. There is little that need or can be done to prevent spread from source cases of chickenpox *or* shingles.

Shingles, being a reactivation of latent virus, is preventible only in those who have not suffered the primary disease, chickenpox.

Patients undergoing immunosuppressive therapy, e.g. children with acute lymphoblastic leukaemia, who suffer chickenpox, suffer more severely and indeed fatal cases occur. Therefore when such immunosuppressed individuals are known to have been in contact with varicella or zoster infection passive immunization with convalescent (high titre) immunoglobulin may modify or prevent infection.

EPSTEIN-BARR VIRUS

The E-B virus is a herpesvirus associated with Burkitt's lymphoma, a malignant tumour occurring only in children and only in certain parts of Africa. Epidemiological evidence suggests a probable insect transmission but a cause and effect relationship has yet to be established and the presence of E-B virus antibodies in many other populations where the tumour is unknown implies that other factors must at least participate in tumour production.

INFECTIOUS MONONUCLEOSIS
(Glandular fever; the Kissing Disease)

Infectious mononucleosis is an acute febrile illness most often seen in young adults and often in epidemic form and antibodies to E-B virus appear in patients suffering infection. Again, when leucocytes from patients with infectious mononucleosis are cultured they give cell lines that contain E-B virus and such cell lines do not develop when leucocytes from uninfected people are cultured. Further proof of a cause and effect relationship between E-B virus and infectious mononucleosis is offered by accidental transmission of the infection when blood from a person incubating the disease is transfused to a healthy individual who then suffers infection.

CHAPTER 31
Orthomyxoviruses

INFLUENZA

Although influenza is not so spectacular as smallpox as a cause of death its spread in a community is faster than any other communicable disease and every 30–40 years pandemic spread across the globe re-affirms this marked capacity of influenza viruses for rapid spread.

Typically influenza is a short sharp febrile illness lasting 2–4 days and the temperature may be alarmingly high, the patient prostrated and toxaemic; symptoms referable to the respiratory tract are usually of a minor nature and the patient's main complaint is of muscle pain and headache and this is perhaps surprising since infection is almost invariably limited to the respiratory epithelium. Patients are infectious to others for only a few days and the virus survives in the environment for only a week or so and is readily destroyed by a variety of disinfectants; hence symptomless or subclinical cases may play an important role in maintaining the virus between epidemic episodes. Infection is acquired by inhalation of droplets from the respiratory secretions of the source case.

Orthomyxoviruses
There are three types, A, B and C, of influenza virus, but they are morphologically identical and the size of the spherical particles is approximately 100nm; they also appear as filamentous forms several microns in length. The capsid is enclosed in a lipid envelope derived from the host cell and from the envelope there project haemagglutinin spikes which confer the haemagglutinating properties on orthomyxoviruses and are active against RBCs of various species. The viruses are sensitive to ether and grow in the amniotic cavity of the chick embryo and in monkey kidney tissue culture.

The three types, A, B and C, can be differentiated from each other by virtue of different complement fixing antigens; type A strains are essentially implicated as the cause of epidemic influenza, type C strains are of doubtful pathogenicity to man and type B strains are usually isolated from clinically mild forms of infection.

Laboratory diagnosis

Microscopy
This is not normally undertaken for diagnosis but immunofluorescent methods are available for detection of virus in specimens of host tissue cells.

Cultivation
Throat washings in saline or a throat swab should be taken to the laboratory immediately for processing or alternatively placed in a transport medium and preserved in a frozen state until received by the laboratory.

Monkey kidney tissue cultures are inoculated, and since a CPE is slight the presence of virus is detected by noting haemadsorption of human group-O RBCs; material should also be inoculated into the amniotic cavity of chick embryos and the virus is detected after 2–3 days incubation by noting agglutination of RBCs. The type of virus present is determined by testing respectively for inhibition of haemadsorption or haemagglutination using specific antisera.

Serology
Influenza may be diagnosed by demonstrating a significant rise in the titre of antibodies between a specimen of serum taken during the acute illness and one obtained 10 days after recovery. Complement fixation tests using the 'S' or soluble antigen (ribonucleoprotein antigen) will show whether the infection was caused by a type A or B virus since the S antigen possessed by all strains of type A virus is identical but different from the S antigen of strains of type B.

Control of influenza
The speed with which the virus spreads combined with the very short incubation period renders unrealistic the isolation of cases in an attempt to prevent epidemic spread.

Active immunization with vaccines which are epidemiologically relevant offers a moderate degree of protection, and immunization should be advocated for key groups at special risk, e.g. nursing and medical personnel; a vaccine is epidemiologically relevant when its antigenic make-up is identical, or almost so, to the epidemic strain in a community.

The speed with which the viruses spread is rivalled only by the ease with which they—especially type A—can undergo antigenic variation so that at any time, stocks of influenza vaccine may be useless in preventing the spread of a new variant.

Antibiotics have no place in the treatment of the primary viral illness but a small proportion of cases, particularly older people and those with predisposing disease, e.g. chronic bronchitis, are prone to bronchopneumonia with pneumococci, staphylococci, *H. influenzae* or *Strept. pyogenes* as the secondary bacterial invader and in such cases prompt and correct antibiotic therapy can be life-saving.

CHAPTER 32
Paramyxoviruses

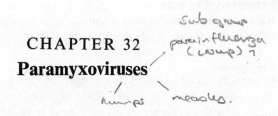

MUMPS, MEASLES, CROUP

The most readily recognized clinical infections in man caused by viruses designated as paramyxoviruses are mumps and measles; certain serotypes, often referred to as the parainfluenza viruses, are the commonest cause of viral croup (acute laryngo-tracheo-bronchitis) and also cause acute respiratory disease which, in severity, is intermediate between influenza and the common cold.

MUMPS

Although the clinical picture of mumps is of a febrile illness accompanied by swelling of the parotid glands or less commonly the submaxillary glands, the infection is viraemic as is shown by the occurrence of meningoencephalitis, orchitis and pancreatitis; it must be noted that these so-called complications can occur without clinically apparent involvement of the salivary glands. A significant proportion, perhaps 40% of cases are symptomless and such clinically inapparent cases make a significant contribution to the spread of infection. Infection is acquired from infected saliva but mumps is not as infectious as other childhood viral infections such as measles or chickenpox; although mumps occurs mostly in 5–15 year olds, the disease occurs in adults who have previously escaped infection and in such instances the incidence of neurological complications is higher than in childhood.

Immunity is long lasting.

The virus
The virus is a single serological entity and like other paramyxoviruses is larger (170nm) than the orthomyxoviruses; envelope contains

a haemagglutinin. Sensitive to ether and grows in the chick embryo amniotic cavity and in tissue cultures of human embryo and monkey kidney. Poor powers of survival outside the host.

Laboratory diagnosis
Rarely requested in cases presenting with typical involvement of the salivary glands but invaluable in cases of mumps meningitis, etc.

Cultivation
Specimens must be transported speedily or kept at $-70°C$ until they can be processed. Monkey kidney tissue cultures are inoculated and after incubation the presence of mumps virus is readily detected by haem-adsorption of fowl RBCs. Alternatively inoculation of the amniotic cavity of chick embryos may be undertaken and after incubation checked for the appearance of haemagglutinin in the amniotic fluid, but not all inoculated eggs show evidence of infection and also salivary specimens may be toxic in the chick embryo. Again the final identification of the virus is by demonstrating inhibition of haemadsorption or haemagglutination with stock antisera.

Serology
Paired sera, i.e. from the acute and convalescent stages of the patient's illness, are tested to show a significant rise in antibody titre in complement fixation tests. Both the 'S' (soluble) antigen and 'V' (viral) antigen should be tested against the specimens of serum; the S antibody appears within 2–3 days and is at maximum titre by 7–10 days and only at this latter time does the V antibody appear; the latter persists for years whereas S antibody cannot be detected beyond 6–9 months after the illness.

Control
Attempts to prevent the spread of mumps by isolating cases are un-successful because of the significant proportion of symptomless cases combined with the fact that typical cases are infectious for 2–3 days *before* the onset of symptoms.

γ-Globulin, prepared from the sera of people convalescing from mumps, has been assessed as a control measure but the only realistic result appears to be a reduction in the incidence of orchitis; its use may be contemplated, provided a supply is available, when epidemics appear in military camps.

Similarly, vaccines have been prepared and tried with reasonable success but are not advocated for wide use at present.

MEASLES

This is the commonest childhood infection and in Britain occurs endemically with epidemic waves every second year; a characteristic maculo-papular rash associated with a usually high fever follows on a prodromal catarrhal illness and the appearance of Koplik's spots. These latter, which are pathognomonic for measles, appear 2-3 days before the skin rash as minute salt-like grains in the buccal mucosa. The disease is highly infectious and spread is from respiratory secretions particularly during the prodromal illness; virus is rarely recovered after the true skin rash has been in evidence for 48 hours. Immunity following recovery from the natural disease is lifelong.

The virus
The virus is a single serological entity and in size is rather larger than the mumps virus; ether sensitive and grows in human amnion tissue culture with a CPE of characteristic large multinucleate giant cells. Does not survive long in the environment.

Laboratory diagnosis
Because of the characteristic clinical picture laboratory confirmation of the diagnosis is rarely sought, but the virus can be isolated in human amnion tissue culture and antibodies can be detected by several techniques, complement fixation tests being the easiest to perform.

Control
Since cases are most infectious before the skin rash appears and then rapidly lose their infectivity, isolation of the florid case is of little use; however reverse isolation, i.e. to reduce the patient's chances of suffering secondary bacterial infection from an exogenous source may be worth while; such complications usually occur in the respiratory tract.

The risk of encephalitis in measles is estimated to be 1 in 1000 cases but the mortality from the complication is about 50%; for this reason and to protect against the secondary bacterial infections associated with the natural disease, vaccines have been introduced. A single dose of an attenuated live vaccine confers long immunity and is now widely advocated although 5–7% of immunised children suffer a mild febrile illness of short duration.

In countries, e.g. Nigeria, where the natural disease is much more severe, with a higher incidence of serious complications and a significantly greater mortality rate, active immunization must be encouraged.

VIRAL CROUP

In common with several other virus groups, e.g. adenoviruses and rhinoviruses, certain of the paramyxoviruses are incriminated in primary infections of the respiratory tract; these particular paramyxoviruses are known as the parainfluenza viruses.

Parainfluenza viruses are the principal cause of viral croup (acute laryngo-tracheo-bronchitis) which occurs mainly in pre-school children.

Of the 4 serotypes of parainfluenza viruses, type 1 is most commonly associated with croup and serotypes 2 and 3 to a lesser extent; in addition all 4 serotypes have been isolated as the causal agents in bronchopneumonia, bronchitis and minor respiratory tract infections.

The parainfluenza viruses are morphologically similar to other paramyxoviruses and agglutinate human group-O erythrocytes; primary isolation is by growth in human kidney tissue culture since these viruses may not grow in the chick embryo and since not all strains produce a CPE in tissue culture the presence of virus is detected by haemadsorption tests with group-O human RBCs and typed by testing for inhibition of haemadsorption with standard antisera.

CHAPTER 33
Arboviruses

'Arbo' is a contraction of '*arthropod-borne*' and the 250 or more viruses in the group *multiply* in arthropod vectors and these latter rarely suffer disease; nor does man always show clinical evidence of infection and subclinical arbovirus acquisitions can be demonstrated by noting a significant rise in specific antibody to a particular member of the group.

Three groupings of clinical illness due to arboviruses can be recognized (1) *Encephalitis*—often in epidemic form, (2) *Systemic febrile disease*, classically dengue and sand-fly fever and (3) *Haemorrhagic fevers*, classically yellow fever.

Fortunately the only disease caused by an arbovirus which is indigenous in Britain is louping ill, a tick-borne disease in sheep which on rare occasions is also suffered by shepherds or laboratory workers investigating outbreaks.

YELLOW FEVER

The clinical picture varies from a fulminating illness to a mild febrile illness or may even be inapparent; classically, however, after an incubation period of 3–6 days there is an early-phase illness coincident with viraemia and with fever, headache, nausea and vomiting predominating; as in many arbovirus infections there follows a remission in this biphasic infection and then a second phase occurs with renewed pyrexia and symptomatology associated with the presence of the virus in particular tissues, e.g. jaundice, intestinal haemorrhage and toxic nephrosis. The essential pathology is mid-zonal necrosis of the liver.

195

The virus

The virus is a serological entity showing many of the general properties of arboviruses, in particular pathogenicity for suckling mice; when inoculated intracerebrally, mice develop encephalitis and virus is detected in brain emulsions by neutralization tests with specific antiserum.

Laboratory diagnosis

During the early viraemic stage blood serum can be inoculated into suckling mice as indicated above. Thereafter diagnosis depends on demonstrating a significant rise in specific antibody titre in paired specimens of the patient's serum.

Control

Urban yellow fever is readily controlled by anti-mosquito measures which eradicate the vector, *Aëdes aegypti*, responsible for transmission from man to man.

The control of jungle or sylvan yellow fever is much more difficult; here transmission is essentially from monkey to monkey, by a variety of jungle mosquitoes. In sylvan yellow fever man is only incidentally a host by virtue of his occupation, e.g. a forester, although if monkeys raid villages and are bitten by *A. aegypti*, the infection can then be transmitted within the domestic situation.

Yellow fever virus was first isolated in 1927 from a Ghanaian patient, Mr Asibi, and it was from this strain that a non-virulent strain, 17D, was derived 10 years later and provided satisfactory prophylaxis.

Although 17D virus is much less stable than the FN (French neurotropic) attenuated virus vaccine it is safer since post-vaccinial encephalitis is very rare; the FN vaccine should not be used in those under 14 years of age because of the risk of associated encephalitis. Both vaccines are highly efficient in protecting against yellow fever.

CHAPTER 34
Picorna viruses

(1) ENTEROVIRUSES

POLIOMYELITIS; BORNHOLM DISEASE; LYMPHOCYTIC MENINGITIS

Polioviruses, coxsackieviruses and echoviruses are grouped together as enteroviruses since they are all acquired by ingestion, replicate in the alimentary tract and have an affinity for central nervous tissue; the enteroviruses also share many other features which are noted below.

POLIOMYELITIS

The polioviruses (especially type 1 virus) are the most paralytogenic of the enteroviruses, *BUT* it must be appreciated that, even in polio-myelitis, paralysis is a rare event and the vast majority (90% +) of people infected with a poliovirus suffer nothing more than a mild influenza-like illness and indeed many infections remain clinically in-apparent. A minority of infected persons will progress beyond this viraemic illness to suffer lymphocytic meningitis without paralysis and recover, whilst in a very few, perhaps only one person of every 1000 infected with a poliovirus, paralysis of one or more muscle groups occurs. Man is the sole natural host of polioviruses and infection is by the faeco-oral route; whilst infection is highest in pre-school children the incidence and severity of the paralytic form of the illness is higher in adults, and certain factors are now accepted as predisposing to increased severity of the clinical illness; these factors include inocula-tion (particularly with alum-precipitated diphtheria toxoid), tonsil-lectomy, prolonged physical activity and fatigue during the incubation period or in the early viraemic stage of the disease. Again pregnant women are much more liable to a paralytic stage than non-pregnant women.

The polioviruses
These and the other enteroviruses belong to the picorna group (pico = small + RNA). The virions are icosahedral, resistant to ether and stable at a low pH (e.g. pH 3); the viruses grow readily in tissue culture, e.g. monkey kidney and human amnion—a tremendous advance on earlier days when the only means of isolation was by inoculating monkeys. The polioviruses are *not* pathogenic for suckling mice, cf. coxsackie-viruses, and three serotypes can be identified by neutralization tests in tissue cultures. Since the introduction of orally administered live attenuated poliovirus vaccine the isolation of a poliovirus from a faecal specimen cannot be assumed to be that of a wild, virulent strain.

Laboratory diagnosis
Specimens of faeces or throat swabs are inoculated on to monkey kidney and human amnion tissue culture, and observed for a CPE. The serotype of the isolate is determined by neutralization tests with standard type-specific antisera.

Differentiation of isolates which may be either wild or attenuated vaccine strains is by inoculation of a monkey in which only the former will display virulence; however, vaccine strains of types 1 and 2 possess several stable marker characteristics which allow their differentiation from wild strains of the same type by *in vitro* methods.

Control
The increasing use of efficient vaccines for active immunization has eliminated endemic poliomyelitis in several countries including Britain. Live attenuated trivalent vaccine (Sabin-type) is given orally as three doses with an interval of 8 weeks between the first and second doses and the third dose is given 4 months after the second dose; this live vaccine gives good protection and is much more easily administered than the earlier inactivated trivalent vaccine (Salk-type) which must be inoculated.

BORNHOLM DISEASE

Synonyms are epidemic myalgia or pleurodynia and the infection, first clearly described in 1933 after an epidemic on the Danish island of

Bornholm, is characterized by fever, severe attacks of muscle pains in the lower thorax and upper abdomen—severe and often sudden in onset and colloquially known as the 'devil's grip'. This is but one of the clinical manifestations caused by coxsackieviruses which are also implicated in herpangina, hand, foot and mouth disease, lymphocytic meningitis, encephalitis, myocarditis and pericarditis, as well as colds and other respiratory infections.

Coxsackieviruses
These are very similar to other enteroviruses, but in addition they are pathogenic to *suckling* mice and hamsters but cannot infect such animals if they are 5 days old or more. Two groups, A and B, of coxsackieviruses are recognized by their affect on suckling mice; intraperitoneal inoculation with group A serotypes results in myositis with *flaccid* paralysis. When group B serotypes are similarly inoculated the resulting myositis produces tremors and *spastic* paralysis and in addition they cause necrosis in the brown fat lobules particularly in the interscapular and cervical pads. Experimental inoculation of Group A strains produces signs of infection much more quickly (4–5 days) than is the case when Group B strains are involved (10 days +). Thirty serotypes are recognized, 24 in Group A and 6 in Group B, by cross neutralization and other tests.

Laboratory diagnosis
Specimens are dealt with as for the isolation of polioviruses but in addition suckling mice are inoculated intraperitoneally; this extra procedure is particularly important in the isolation of Group A viruses which do not grow well in tissue culture.

Control
The virtually universal presence of the coxsackieviruses in the intestinal tract and the ease with which they can be spread by the faeco-oral route has denied any attempts at control.

LYMPHOCYTIC MENINGITIS

Lymphocytic meningitis is a term used to contrast with pyogenic meningitis since the CSF in the former is clear in appearance and the lymphocyte predominates. Synonyms for lymphocytic meningitis are aseptic meningitis and viral meningitis, but the latter is a misnomer since certain bacteria can produce a similar syndrome.

The opportunity is taken here, however, of considering briefly the role of enteroviruses in lymphocytic meningitis since it is a common manifestation of enteroviral infection. It has already been mentioned that infection with polioviruses may produce lymphocytic meningitis and all 6 serotypes of Group B coxsackieviruses and a few types of Group A are also implicated. Similarly 20 of the 33 recognized serotypes of echoviruses have been implicated in epidemics and sporadic cases of lymphocytic meningitis. It must be stressed that lymphocytic meningitis is only one form of clinical expression of enteroviral infection and, for example, in the domestic situation when a case occurs, other members of the family may suffer inapparent infection with the same serotype or may suffer a non-meningeal febrile illness perhaps with a rash.

Echoviruses
These are very similar to the polio and coxsackieviruses but unlike the latter are without pathogenicity for suckling mice although one type (type 9) produces a coxsackie Group A response after several passages in tissue culture.

Laboratory diagnosis
This is by isolation by the methods used for polioviruses.

(2) RHINOVIRUSES

THE COMMON COLD

These viruses, like the enteroviruses, belong to the picorna group and are the agents mainly responsible for that most common and recurring of human infections. Although the common cold is experienced more frequently in the colder months in temperate climates the infection occurs throughout the world and there is no evidence that exposure to low temperatures in any way predisposes to infection. Hardly without exception the infection is short-lived although pharyngitis with a dry cough may persist for several days after the cold itself has disappeared.

Extension of inflammation to the middle ear and the nasal sinuses is common and similarly secondary bacterial infection may occur with prolongation of disease.

The viruses
These belong to the picorna group but are inactivated at acid pH which the enteroviruses can tolerate; otherwise they share most of the

characteristics of enteroviruses. Three groups of rhinoviruses are distinguished according to the tissue culture which gives optimal growth; the M group prefer monkey kidney, the H group grow only in human embryo cells and O group strains grow only in organ culture. Members of the M and H groups require to be grown at 33°C. There are at least 55 serotypes of rhinoviruses.

Laboratory diagnosis
This is very rarely sought in the common cold although the viruses can be isolated from nasal or mouth washings when inoculated on human embryo kidney cells incubated at 33°C. Serotype identification of the isolation is by neutralization tests with standard antisera.

Control
Control is virtually impossible.

CHAPTER 35
Hepatitis viruses

INFECTIOUS HEPATITIS, SERUM HEPATITIS

Although hepatitis is a feature of many bacterial and viral infections, e.g. leptospirosis and yellow fever, there are two distinct syndromes which merit special consideration since *inter alia* they have particular clinical and epidemiological significance.

INFECTIOUS HEPATITIS (Virus A)

Many cases, particularly in children, are mild and may be so slight as to escape medical attention. Classically the symptoms are those of obstructive jaundice with nausea, malaise, slight fever; the stools are pale and the urine dark. Infection is usually by ingestion and follows after an incubation period of 2–6 weeks; faeco-oral spread is from cases and carriers and on occasion the vehicle may be water contaminated by sewage or shellfish which have fed in sewage-contaminated waters and are then eaten without adequate cooking. Since there is a viraemic phase in infectious hepatitis it is always possible for blood from a subclinical case of infection to be transfused and cause the disease in the recipient but this is an uncommon method of spread in infectious hepatitis.

Infectious hepatitis is endemic throughout the world, epidemics occur during the colder months of the year and are more common in rural than in urban communities; most common in the first two decades of life. Mortality is low.

SERUM HEPATITIS (Virus B)

Apart from the insidious onset of serum hepatitis compared with the usually abrupt manner in which infectious hepatitis declares itself, the clinical manifestations of the two infections are very similar, hence the need for taking a full and careful history from the patient particularly in regard to association with other cases of jaundice. The incubation period of serum hepatitis is long—2–6 months or more; spread is essentially by parenteral inoculation and many cases are iatrogenic, e.g. following blood transfusion or administration of blood products, communal use of styletes or syringes at diabetic, haematology or venereology clinics or at immunization centres. Indeed every injection must be regarded as a hazard both to patient and practitioner! Tattooing has been implicated as an efficient means of acquiring serum hepatitis and drug addicts are also at risk and the amount of blood required to be inoculated is so small—0·01 ml or less—that infection can be transmitted through superficial scratches from twigs and bushes contaminated from carriers; this hazard was noted among track runners in Sweden. Infection is sporadic although epidemics have occurred, e.g. in renal dialysis units; there is no special seasonal incidence and no age group is particularly involved. Serum hepatitis tends to be a more severe infection than infectious hepatitis and certainly has a higher mortality rate.

The viruses
Until recently most of our knowledge of the viruses had been acquired by studying the infections in human volunteers and in particular their separate identities had been shown by demonstrating the homologous nature of immunity following natural infection. An antigen, known as Australia antigen (synonyms include Hepatitis B antigen (HB ag), SH antigen) has been demonstrated in the blood of cases and carriers of serum hepatitis; electron microscopy of Australia antigen, from the serum of cases and carriers reveals particles of a size between 20 and 45nm. As yet no antigen has been seen in the blood or faeces of individuals suffering or recovered from infectious hepatitis. Other factors, e.g. resistance of both viruses to ether and their relative thermostability (tolerate 60°C for 4 hr) have been demonstrated in infection experiments with human volunteers but a more complete knowledge of the viruses must await their isolation in pure form in tissue culture and other systems.

Laboratory diagnosis
With the exception of demonstrating Australia antigen, e.g. by immunoelectroosmophoresis, or its antibody by radioimmunoassay, laboratory diagnosis is essentially by elimination of other possible

infective causes of hepatitis. Thus specimens of faeces should be examined for enteroviruses, a blood-film examined and total and differential white cell counts made for a possible diagnosis of infectious mononucleosis and paired serum samples should be screened for significant antibody rise against other hepatitogenic agents, e.g. leptospirae, adenoviruses, enteroviruses, etc.

Control
Preventive measures for infectious hepatitis include those used to reduce spread of faeco-orally acquired infections and in addition gamma globulin offers short-lived passive immunity. However, gamma globulin preparations have little or no protective influence in serum hepatitis but iatrogenic episodes can be dramatically reduced by screening blood for transfusion or use in dialysis units and any blood containing Australia antigen rejected; similarly the use of disposable syringes and needles and styletes helps to reduce spread of Virus B. These elementary precautions must be strictly observed since it is not only those suffering and recovering from a clinically declared attack of serum hepatitis who are a source of infection; a proportion of apparently healthy individuals, e.g. 1 in every 800 blood donors, possesses Australia antigen!

CHAPTER 36
Rhabdoviruses

RABIES

Although rhabdoviruses cause disease in plants, insects and are also responsible for bovine vesicular stomatitis the most significant infection is rabies; rabies occurs naturally in a wide variety of mammals both domestic, e.g. dogs, cats and farm animals, and wild, e.g. skunks, foxes and several types of bat. Man is infected when bitten by a rabid animal or when saliva from the animal contaminates a skin scratch or abrasion; the incubation period to the onset of symptoms may be only 4 weeks if the bite is on the head or neck or as long as 12 weeks if on a lower limb. Longer incubation periods are known—even up to two years. The virus is carried from the infection site to the CNS via the nerves. Symptoms include fever and headache; difficulty in swallowing, so-called hydrophobia, is only one evidence of muscle contractions. Generalized convulsions follow with delirium and a fatal outcome is inevitable.

The virus
There is only one serotype of this RNA virus which is bullet-shaped and measures 75×180nm. The virus grows well in tissue culture, e.g. of hamster kidney and in chick embryos; it is pathogenic for mice and other experimental animals and in nerve tissue, particularly in the hippocampus, produces Negri bodies which are pathognomonic for rabies. Negri bodies are multiple eosinophilic cytoplasmic inclusions measuring from 0·5 to 20μm.

Laboratory diagnosis
In areas where rabies is known to occur the patient's history and the clinical picture usually suffice without recourse to the laboratory.

However, specimens of saliva, CSF and urine can be used to inoculate mice intracerebrally and after an increasing flaccid paralysis the animal dies in 7–14 days, and the demonstration of Negri bodies clinches the diagnosis. Negri bodies can also be noted post mortem in the human case and the virus can be demonstrated by immunofluorescence.

Control

Some countries are free from rabies, e.g. Britain, Australia and New Zealand, but only because of strict quarantine rules for importation of animals. Control of the natural infection in domestic animals is relatively easy, e.g. the number of cases of rabies in dogs in America has dropped from over 5000 in 1953 to only 180 in 1973. On the other hand rabies in wild animals is virtually impossible to eradicate and indeed the incidence in some species, e.g. bats, has risen very significantly in America in the last 20 years.

Specific prevention is possible even in the individual bitten by a rabid animal since the long incubation period of the disease allows active immunity to be conferred by artificial means.

Two vaccines are available but must be given daily for 14 consecutive days—an uncomfortable prospect but preferable to the inevitability of death. The Semple vaccine is of phenol-inactivated virus from infected rabbit brain but carries a slight risk of allergic encephalomyelitis caused by repeated injection of nerve tissue; another vaccine for human use is derived from infected duck embryos and its use eliminates the risk of encephalomyelitis—it is stated to be slightly less protective than the Semple vaccine.

CHAPTER 37
Rubella

Rubella or German measles is a mild, essentially uncomplicated, short-lived childhood fever with a macular rash, some degree of pharyngitis and enlargement of the cervical lymph glands. This essentially trivial illness shot into prominence in 1941 when on clinical and epidemiological grounds it was observed that infection occurring in the early months of pregnancy resulted in the offspring suffering congenital cataract often accompanied by cardiac defects.

The teratogenic properties of the rubella virus are now recognized and it is estimated that when mothers suffer rubella in the first month of pregnancy approximately half of the offspring will show defects, if the infection is contracted in the 2nd, 3rd or 4th month the estimated proportion of children suffering defects is 25%, 17% and 11%. The main defects are deafness, cardiac defects, e.g. patent ductus arteriosus and cataract; the earlier in pregnancy that rubella occurs the greater the risk of multiple defects if the child survives to term. The incidence of stillbirths and prematurity is also increased in women who suffer rubella in the first 16 weeks of pregnancy.

The virus
A lesser reason than its teratogenic properties for considering the rubella virus separately is that its taxonomic position is not yet defined. Apparently there is only one serotype of this RNA virus and it is ether-sensitive, agglutinates erythrocytes from day-old chicks and grows in various tissue cultures but produces a CPE only in the rabbit kidney cell line, RK13.

Laboratory diagnosis
This is rarely requested except when a pregnant woman is thought to be suffering infection; during the acute phase of the illness the virus can

207

be recovered by tissue culture of material taken from a throat swab and as well as noting the CPE, immunofluorescent techniques will detect the virus in the tissue culture cells. Since the pregnant woman exposed to rubella may suffer an inapparent infection, paired sera should be checked by the haemagglutination-inhibition technique to determine the presence of rubella antibodies and to demonstrate whether or not there is a significant rise in antibody titre.

Control

No interest in preventing rubella was shown until it was known that the virus could interfere with organogenesis in the human embryo; thereafter passive immunization with gamma globulin prepared from pooled human sera was used but with variable and in the main doubtful protective benefit. Active immunization with a single dose of live, attenuated vaccine is most efficient and should be given to girls at puberty; the vaccine *should not be given* to pregnant women or women who may become pregnant in the following 6–8 weeks.

PROTOZOOLOGY AND MYCOLOGY

CHAPTER 38
Protozoology

Although protozoa are unicellular microscopic organisms which, like bacteria, can cause disease in human and other hosts their resemblance to bacteria is only slight. In cellular organization protozoa are much more close to animal cells since their nuclei are similar, cell division is virtually identical and food is ingested and then digested intracellularly.

Again, unlike bacteria most protozoa show complex life cycles with different morphological forms and protozoa are unaffected by antibiotics which in similar concentrations have antibacterial effects.

Protozoal infections occur throughout the world but the more severe diseases occur mainly outside temperate zones so that Britain is free of many such except occasional imported cases; such imported cases rarely act as sources of infection within this country since, e.g. in the case of malaria, conditions necessary for transmission do not exist.

MALARIA

Man can only naturally suffer malaria when he is bitten by the vector, i.e. female anopheline mosquitoes which are the definitive hosts for the infecting plasmodia. The genus *Plasmodium* comprises many species which can parasitize reptiles, birds and mammals, but man can only be infected with four species, *P. falciparum*, *P. malariae*, *P. ovale* and *P. vivax* and although heroic malaria eradication campaigns, launches by the World Health Organization, have influenced the incidence of malaria, this disease remains a major cause of ill health in many parts of the world and is thus also economically important.

Schizogony is the term used for the asexual cycle in the life of pladmodia and occurs in the human (or other) intermediate host after he is bitten by a parasitized definitive host, the female anopheline mosquito.

The infective form of the malarial parasite, the sporozoite, is slender and spindle-shaped with a single nucleus; from the bite-site sporozoites must gain access to liver parenchymal cells since only there can primary schizogony occur.

In schizogony the nucleus of the plasmodial cell divides repeatedly within an expanding cytoplasm and cytoplasmic fission is delayed until growth stops; thereafter thousands of small single-nucleus merozoites are liberated into the blood stream and, with the exception of *P. falciparum*, can also invade fresh liver cells to produce a continuing exo-erythrocytic cycle. The merozoites produced during this pre-erythrocytic hepatic cycle, which occupies 5–15 days depending on the species of plasmodium, then invade red blood cells to establish an erythrocytic cycle during which the merozoite feeds on the protein portion of haemoglobin; a central vacuole appears within the merozoite shortly after entering the RBC to give a ringform appearance to the parasite and after a few hours of growth and feeding the trophozoite fills the entire RBC. Nuclear fission follows to produce the erythrocytic schizont with the ultimate production of some 5–24 merozoites which escape when the RBC ruptures and these can then attack fresh RBCs or be ingested by a mosquito taking a blood meal.

Erythrocytic schizogony is of 48 hr duration (72 hr in the case of *P. malariae*) and the outpouring of merozoites from the RBCs is coincidental with recurring bouts of fever. Gametocytes, i.e. sexual forms, are also produced in RBCs and their further development is dependent on ingestion by the mosquito host.

Sporogony: Although this sexual stage in the life of the plasmodium begins in the human host with the production of the gametocytes, its fulfilment takes place in the mosquito's stomach once the sexual forms are released from the ingested RBCs. Development of the liberated microgametocyte (male) is known appropriately as exflagellation and following three consecutive divisions of the nucleus eight highly motile flagella-like structures form at the cell surface and these microgametes then break from the cell and thrash about in the mosquito's stomach. Simultaneously the female form (the macrogametocyte) matures to a macrogamete by forming polar bodies and is then ready for fertilization by a motile microgamete. The resultant zygote becomes crescent-shaped and motile (the oökinete) which invades the stomach epithelium and establishes itself under the basement membrane on the outer surface of the mosquito's stomach. Here numerous oökinetes can settle and then assume a non-motile, rounded shape, the oöcyst; during the next 10–14 days the final stage of sporogony occurs with the production of thousands of sporozoites which are liberated into the coelom whence the vast majority migrate to penetrate the salivary glands and await injection into a susceptible human host to allow another cycle of schizogony to take place.

Laboratory diagnosis
The microscopic examination of blood films stained by Leishman's or some other Romanowsky stain is the basis of laboratory diagnosis; thick blood films can be rapidly scanned for the presence of malaria parasites and then examination of a thin blood film allows identification of the particular species of plasmodia.

Species identification depends on differences in the size, shape and arrangement of the merozoites, trophozoites and gametocytes as well as varying changes effected in the host RBC.

Prevention
Obvious measures include the treatment of cases and eradication of the vector mosquitoes, e.g. by eliminating breeding places in swamps and smaller collections of water; similarly protection of human hosts from bites by screening premises and using mosquito nets and insect repellants is essential. Chemoprophylaxis, e.g. with proguanil for those living in or visiting areas where malaria is endemic is an added preventive measure.

AMOEBIASIS

The causal organism is *Entamoeba histolytica* and it is parasitic on man and other primates. The organism exists in two forms; the vegetative or trophozoite form normally lives in the colon and may exist there for months or even years without causing symptoms of disease. The cyst form also occurs in the human gut but unlike the trophozoite can survive outside the host's body, and it is this latter form which is transmitted from one individual to another. Factors which are known to precipitate infection include malnutrition in general and avitaminosis in particular. Similarly, infection may declare itself when another infection, e.g. bacillary dysentery, acts as a triggering mechanism. Amoebiasis usually presents as dysenteric illness in which shallow ulcers form in the intestinal mucosa and the patient's symptoms are those of chronic diarrhoeal disease with blood and mucus present in the stool. On the other hand, amoebae may spread either by direct extension within the bowel wall or by blood spread usually to the liver with amoebic abscess formation. Involvement of other tissues may occur but it is unusual. It should be noted that cysts are never found in tissue lesions.

Epidemiology
The fragility of the trophozoite which dies very rapidly outside the host, explains why it is rarely the infecting agent; the cyst forms which develop from the trophozoite in the large bowel and are excreted in the faeces can survive for days and epidemic spread can take place if cystic forms pollute a water supply. Hand to mouth spread by cysts from a case or, more often, a carrier can easily occur by fouling of vegetables and other foodstuffs.

Laboratory diagnosis
The laboratory diagnosis depends primarily on the demonstration of trophozoites and/or cysts in the faeces and where a search for trophozoites is to be made the stool specimen must be examined within one hour of being passed. Ideally, microscopy of a wet film should be carried out immediately the stool is obtained. The characteristics of the trophozoites are those of any amoeba and the presence of red blood cells within the amoeba is diagnostic of its pathogenic nature. *Ent. histolytica* is larger than other commensal amoeba which may occur in the human gut and the nucleus contains a centrally situated karyosome and a ring of fine chromatin granules lying on the nuclear membrane.

The cyst forms which can be concentrated by the simple zinc sulphate flotation technique are spherical, only half the size (10–20μm) of the trophozoite and the cyst has a single smooth wall and is transluscent. Internally one or two refractile bodies may be seen and these are known as chromatoid bodies or chromidial bars which are reserves of ribonucleoprotein. The cysts of *Ent. histolytica* may resemble those of other lumen dwelling protozoa but where more than 4 nuclei are noted, the cysts are not those of *Ent. histolytica*.

GIARDIASIS

Infection with *Giardia lamblia*, a flagellate protozoon, is world wide in comparison with a restriction of amoebic infection to tropical and subtropical zones. Giardial infection occurs, usually in epidemic form in Britain, amongst children and particularly those in residential institutions. The organism occurs both as a trophozoite and also in a cyst form and it is the latter, excreted in faeces, which can be transmitted to a fresh host, usually by poor personal hygiene and therefore by the hand-to-mouth route. Infection even when it occurs epidemically is frequently not thought of until bacterial causes have been eliminated.

Laboratory diagnosis
Freshly passed faecal specimens should be examined as wet films for the trophozoite stage and these have a unique rolling movement; in stained preparations two nuclei lying side by side in the broader anterior end of the cell can be noted.

Cysts are best examined after the specimen has been concentrated by the zinc sulphate flotation method. Cysts are pear-shaped, refractile bodies with a double wall and a diametrically placed axostyle is usually evident.

TRICHOMONIASIS

Numerous species of trichomonads are recognized and given specific names associated with the host which is parasitized, but the organisms are morphologically identical whether the host is human, canine, feline or simian. Cysts are not formed. The organisms associated with the human host are named *Trichomonas vaginalis* when they occur in the genitourinary system and *T. hominis* when observed in the faeces, but there is immunological evidence to suggest that these are in fact separate species. Surveys of healthy individuals reveal that Trichomonads can exist in an apparently commensal state in the sites at which they occasionally declare their pathogenicity, i.e. the vagina, the urethra and prostate; with very few exceptions, infection is transmitted by sexual intercourse and even then, symptoms may be few or even absent. In the female trichomonas vaginitis frequently co-exists with gonorrhoea or moniliasis and indeed the diagnosis of gonorrhoea may be difficult to make until the trichomonad infection has been treated.

Laboratory diagnosis
Microscopy of wet film preparations is usually the only procedure undertaken but media suitable for culturing trichomonads are available.

CHAPTER 39
Mycology

Introduction

The vast majority of fungi are saprophytes and thus participate in the deomposition of plant and animal wastes; additionally fungi, by contaminating culture media and foodstuffs, can irritate man and although fungal disease in plants is common only a few are pathogenic to man and animals. A few fungi are therapeutically valuable to man since they are a source of antibacterial agents.

Less than 100 of the thousands of fungi recognized have been associated with human disease and most fungal infections are of body surfaces, the *superficial mycoses*, and occur throughout the world regardless of climate and race, e.g. ringworm.

Deep-seated or generalized fungal infections, the *systemic mycoses*, are less common and their incidence differs from country to country, e.g. they are rare in Britain but common in some American States.

Furthermore inhalation of the spores of some otherwise non-pathogenic species of fungi can precipitate allergic reactions in the human host.

Classification of fungi

A formal classification of fungi, made primarily on the nature of their sexual processes, defines four classes, but since the sexual stages are rarely seen a more practical classification into four morphological groups offers an intelligent nomenclature for their identification and for communication among applied mycologists and to clinicians.

The first group comprises the MOULDS which grow as branching filaments (hyphae) which intermingle and form a dense, felted mass (the mycelium); the *vegetative* mycelium grows into the surface of the substrate and absorbs foodstuffs whereas the *aerial* mycelium projects

214

into the air and from its hyphae, sexual spores develop which are shed into the environment.

YEASTS comprise the second morphological group; these uni-cellular fungi which appear as round or ovoid cells, do not form sexual spores but reproduce by budding of the parent cell. On solid media yeast colonies are similar to those of staphylococci and thus contrast with the fluffy colonies of the moulds.

The third group, the YEAST-LIKE FUNGI, also reproduce by budding and grow either as round or ovoid cells or as non-branching filaments (pseudo hyphae); colonies of the yeast-like fungi resemble those of bacteria.

Finally the DIMORPHIC FUNGI acquired their title since they grow as yeast forms in tissues or when incubated at 37°C *in vitro*; contrarily when cultures are grown at 22°C they appear as a mycelial growth.

Laboratory identification

Microscopy

Microscopy plays a more important part in the identification of genera and species of fungi than it does in the bacterial world; so much so that microscopy of either unstained or stained preparations of specimens from lesions or from resultant cultures is usually sufficient for an identification to be made.

Skin scales, hair or nail clippings from cases of tinea (ringworm) must be rendered transparent, i.e. 'cleared' before the infecting fungi can be seen and clearing is achieved by immersing the specimen in 20% sodium or potassium hydroxide. The specimen is usually placed on a microscope slide, covered with the clearing reagent and a coverslip applied; the preparation is left at room temperature to allow the keratin to be partially dissolved—this manœuvre takes 5–10 min except for nail specimens which may have to be treated for 1–3 hr at 37°C. With such specimens it is better to immerse the nail clippings in a tube containing 20% NaOH (or KOH) so that digestion can proceed without having to replenish the agent frequently on a slide preparation.

When digestion of the keratin is complete, excess NaOH is removed by pressing gently on the coverslip with blotting paper so that the thin film of material can be examined with the dry objectives; staining of the preparation is with lactophenol blue applied at one interface between coverslip and slide and the hydroxide removed from the opposing interface with blotting paper.

Material from suspected cases of candidosis can be stained by Gram's method as can cultures obtained from such specimens and wet film India ink preparations are used to demonstrate the capsules of *Cryptococcus neoformans* in cerebrospinal fluid or material from animals experimentally infected with that agent.

Cultivation

Sabouraud's glucose peptone agar is the medium most commonly employed in the isolation of fungi; the pH of this medium is 5·4 and parallel cultivation on the basic medium with the addition of thiamine enhances spore formation by some ringworm fungi. Incubation is under aerobic conditions at 28°C and because of the slow growth of many fungal species plates are retained for three weeks although many positive cultures will be visible within a few days and growth sufficiently advanced for identification by 1–2 weeks.

Not only should the characteristics of the surface growth be noted but the appearances of the undersurface of the colony and the presence of pigments which may or may not diffuse into the medium greatly assist identification of the species; microscopic examination of the sporing mycelium in a *needle mount preparation* confirms identification by allowing the recognition of the size, shape and distribution of micro- and macro-conidia. Such preparations involve the removal of a portion of the mycelium which is then teased out in a drop of 95% ethyl alcohol on the surface of a microscope slide; a drop of lactophenol blue stain is applied just before the alcohol has evaporated and then a coverslip is applied, the stain is allowed to penetrate for a few minutes at room temperature and after blotting over the coverslip to remove excess stain, the preparation is viewed with low and high power dry objectives.

Slide culture technique

This method allows microscopic examination of growing mycelium to be made intermittently and without disturbing the growth; a block of sterile Sabouraud's agar is held between a sterile slide and coverslip. The agar block is inoculated at each of the vertical sides and then incubated in a closed chamber, e.g. a plastic sandwich box at 28°C; humid conditions are maintained by placing in the chamber several layers of blotting paper soaked in 20% glycerol.

Intermittent microscopic examination can be made without disturbing the preparation and as soon as adequate sporing is noted lactophenol blue preparations can be made from material on the slide and the undersurface of the coverslip. Such stained preparations can be rendered permanent by sealing, e.g. with nail varnish, the slide with a fresh coverslip and vice versa.

DERMATOPHYTIC FUNGI

RINGWORM

Tinea, or ringworm, are superficial infections restricted to the keratinous layers of the skin, hairs or nails caused by three genera, *Microsporum*, *Trichophyton* and *Epidermophyton*; although such infections do not extend below the keratinous layer, skin lesions spread outwards to produce ring-like lesions with an active infected edge which is vesicular or perhaps pustular while the central healing lesion becomes dusky, dry and scaly.

Certain species of ringworm fungi are primarily *anthrophilic* whereas others are essentially *zoophilic*, causing similar infections in animals whence human hosts may be infected, e.g. from household pets or farm animals. Again, some species, e.g. *Trichophyton mentagrophytes*, can cause infection in skin, hair or nails, whereas others, e.g. *Microsporum* species, commonly incriminated in scalp ringworm (tinea capitis) do not affect nails.

When zoophilic species infect humans the lesions are usually more severe than those produced by anthrophilic species of dermatophytic fungi.

Laboratory diagnosis

Specimens may be contaminated with commensal bacteria or with pathogenic species acting as secondary invaders therefore skin scrapings, nail clippings or affected hairs should be taken only after the affected area has been cleansed with 70% alcohol to reduce the bacterial population. Specimens should be submitted in individual containers and clearly marked for identification.

Microscopic examination

This is made of unstained or of lactophenol blue stained preparations after the specimen has been cleared with hydroxide and with specimens of hair note should be taken of whether the infection is endothrix or ectothrix and whether the spores are of the small or large type.

Cultivation

The specimen should be treated with 78% alcohol for 2–3 min to reduce bacterial contamination and then fragments of the specimen are implanted into the surface of a plate of Sabouraud's agar. Incubation is under aerobic conditions and at 28°C; the plates are examined every 3 days and fungal growth spreads outwards from the site of implantation so that if subculture, e.g. to slide culture, is undertaken the inoculum should be from the edge of the developing colony to avoid the growth of any contaminating bacteria.

Identification of species depends on noting the speed of growth, the surface appearance of the colony and the appearance of its undersurface as well as the presence of pigments; as already noted, needle mount preparations of the aerial mycelium, stained with lactophenol blue and examined microscopically reveal the presence of micro- and/or macro-conidia. The morphology of these latter characterizes the three genera.

Microsporum species produce large, thick-walled, fusiform conidia, each divided into numerous cells by transverse septa; microconidia are not commonly seen in *Microsporum* species and then only in small numbers. *M. audouinii* does not produce conidia when grown on Sabouraud's medium and the growth comprises only interlacing hyphae.

Trichophyton species when grown on Sabouraud's medium are characterized by the abundance of microconidia which are spherical and borne singly from the sides of the hyphae; macroconidia are rarely seen but when they occur they are cylindrical, small and thin-walled.

Epidermophyton species do not yield microconidia in artificial cultures; they produce thin-walled, finger-like macroconidia which in older cultures become clubbed or pear-shaped.

PATHOGENIC YEAST-LIKE FUNGI

There are many species within the genus *Candida* but only one, *C. albicans*, is commonly encountered as a human pathogen and it is also present as a commensal in the buccal cavity, throat, intestine, vagina and the skin.

Infection is usually localized and superficial and occurs at sites where the organism exists commensally so that the finding of *C. albicans* is not necessarily equated with active infection; candidosis may present as oral thrush in the young infant or as vaginal thrush—particularly in pregnancy. Cutaneous candidosis is normally restricted to the warm moist skin flexures although infection of the hands is an occupational hazard in those whose work requires prolonged immersion in water. The endogenous nature of candidosis is emphasized by the fact that infection is often precipitated when a patient is treated for other infections with broad-spectrum antibiotics which dramatically reduce the population of normal commensal bacteria and open the pathway for *C. albicans* to show its opportunistic pathogenic abilities. Other categories of patients who are predisposed to infection with *C. albicans* include diabetics, alcoholics and drug addicts as well as those receiving corticosteroids or immunosuppressive agents.

C. albicans is a typical yeast-like fungus and the budding yeast cells and long filaments stain Gram-positively and these structures are much larger than bacteria which will also be present in specimens taken from patches of thrush.

Laboratory diagnosis

The organism can be isolated when material from the lesion is plated on blood agar or Sabouraud's medium; colonies are cream-coloured and resemble those of staphylococci and cultures have a characteristic odour.

Differentiation of *C. albicans* from the less frequently encountered species, e.g. *C. stellatoidea* and *C. tropicalis* is best undertaken in a Reference Laboratory.

PATHOGENIC YEASTS

Cryptococcus neoformans is the only pathogenic member of the genus and only rarely can it be recovered from healthy human beings; cryptococcosis occurs sporadically in Britain and usually presents as a chronic meningitis which is preceded by a transient, self-limiting lung infection. Although cryptococcosis may occasionally be endogenous, infection is usually acquired exogenously by inhalation and *C. neoformans* can be isolated from various animals and birds and is present in their excreta and can survive in soil.

Human infection may also result in cutaneous lesions or bone abscesses and granulomas of lymph glands.

Laboratory diagnosis

The *laboratory diagnosis* depends firstly on microscopic examination of CSF or other specimens to demonstrate the characteristic spherical heavily capsulate yeast cells; these are best seen in wet India ink films and budding of some cells will also be noted.

Cultivation of material on Sabouraud's medium yields colonies similar to those of *Staphylococcus albus* after 2 or 3 days at 37°C; on further incubation the colonies become increasingly mucoid and tan coloured.

C. neoformans is the only species within the genus which is pathogenic for mice; following intraperitoneal inoculation with pathological
material or laboratory cultures the animal sickens and dies within 2–3
weeks and post mortem examination reveals gelatinous masses of the
yeasts not only intraperitoneally but in the brain tissue.

Index